Other titles by G. J. Ebrahim include:

Breast Feeding: the Biological Option
Child Care in the Tropics
Child Health in a Changing Environment
Practical Mother and Child Health in Developing Countries
Handbook of Tropical Paediatrics
Paediatric Practice in Developing Countries
Maternal and Child Health Around the World (with Helen Wallace)
Care of the Newborn in Developing Countries
Nutrition in Mother and Child Health

The Authors and Publishers wish to thank CAFOD (The Catholic Fund for Overseas Development) for generously subsidising the paperback edition of this book.

District Health Care

Challenges for Planning, Organisation and Evaluation in Developing Countries

R. Amonoo-Lartson

G. J. Ebrahim

H. J. Lovel

J. P. Ranken

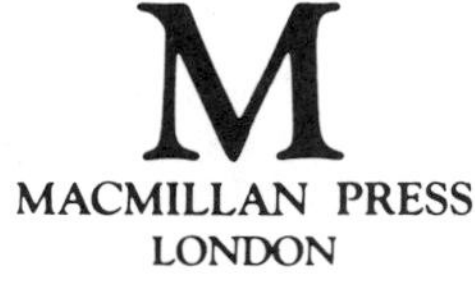

MACMILLAN PRESS
LONDON

First published 1984 by
THE MACMILLAN PRESS LTD
London and Basingstoke
Companies and representatives throughout the world.

Printed in Hong Kong

ISBN 0 333 36600 X   hardcover
ISBN 0 333 36601 8   paperback

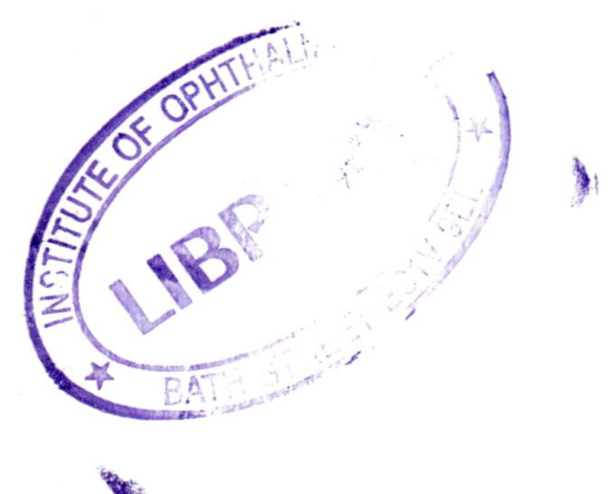

Contents

Preface

In 1961 when I was involved with other colleagues at the Ministry of Health in Tanzania in planning the mother and child health services, we knew very little about management and planning. There was also not much help available from the existing medical literature at the time. All we had was the objective of making basic health care available to the vulnerable groups who together made up two-thirds of Tanzania's population. More than 90 per cent of the country's population was rural, living in widely dispersed homesteads or scattered family groups. There were no models of health care planning which we could follow. Besides there was the growing doubt that many of the modern approaches and concepts in health care had evolved out of the experiences of the Western industrial societies which are predominantly urban and have access to far greater resources than any developing country can ever muster. How relevant would the Western systems of health care be for Tanzania's health problems? Independent Tanzania with a highly committed leadership required basic health care to reach out to all its people, however remotely situated and whatever their social status. A start was made in which all available health resources came to be mobilised with a growing reliance on medical auxiliaries and paramedical personnel. Inevitably many mistakes were made, but they also provided the much-needed learning experience.

For many years it had been my wish to describe the lessons learned from my Tanzanian experience. I knew I lacked the breadth of experience necessary for such a task even though my travels with the WHO/UNICEF-sponsored course, for senior teachers of child health, gave me the opportunity to study the health services of several countries. When Hermione Lovel joined the Tropical Child Health Unit, the idea of this book began to develop further. She had completed a study for Ghana entitled 'Future steps towards a Primary Health Care Strategy for Ghana' and a major part of this book is based on her experience of Ghana's health care problems.

During the period when Hermione Lovel was conducting her enquiry into Ghana's health systems, Dr Amonoo-Lartson was the Chairman of the Primary Health Care sub-committee of the Health Manpower Committee. His special area of interest is management in health. During the period 1977–81 when he was deputy director of Medical Services in Ghana he carried responsibility for the management of the hospital services, including the co-ordination of church-related hospitals with the national health system. He had also been involved in the evaluation of several development projects in Ghana and knew that for Primary Care to succeed, close relationships and support with hospital services were essential. It is not a question of 'either/or', but that both types of health care working together in harmony is essential. Such harmonious relationships require good management.

When John Ranken joined the Tropical Child Health Unit he brought with him not only expertise in management but also the experience of teaching the subject to members of the health and nursing professions. We knew that the four of us could pool our experiences to compile a text for colleagues working in remote areas of the developing world with no access to literature or professional managerial advice.

The book is less than half the size of the material originally compiled by us. There are several topics which need lengthier discussion and several other topics which had to be left out. Considerations of cost have imposed restrictions on the size of the book. However, the cost of the paperback version of the present edition has been kept low because of a generous printing subsidy from CAFOD (The Catholic Fund for Overseas Development) to whom the authors are indebted. In the meantime we would depend on our readers for suggestions and advice concerning future changes.

G. J. EBRAHIM

1 The Need for Management in District Health Care

WHO IS THIS BOOK FOR? IN WHAT DISTRICT

People working at District level in many countries are now frequently faced with the task of putting a national Primary Health Care policy into action. Sometimes detailed plans exist as, for example, in Ghana, the Sudan or India; but in many other countries there is no detailed plan. Many problems are being experienced and the object of this book is to identify the ways in which some of these problems can be tackled. The book is intended for anyone who can identify with any of the issues in table 1.1.

Frequently people experiencing such problems will be members of a District Health Team (DHT). Often some of them will have had a clinical training (for example, as a doctor, a nurse or a nutritionist) and be faced with much non-

Table 1.1 **This book is intended for anyone who can identify with any of the following issues. (Tick if they apply to you.)**

Tick

1 'I'm too busy, I never have time'
2 'We can't do it, there aren't enough midwives'
3 'There aren't enough drugs'
4 'There's no money left to pay transport costs'
5 'It's the fault of the bureaucrats'
6 'I never knew those people had such problems, they never used our services'
7 'We have done so much to expand the services'
8 'I thought our job was just inside the hospital'
9 'There are no people to control all this rubbish'
10 'We're a new team, we don't know what to do'
11 'People don't recognise the work we do'
12 'What could traditional healers do?'
13 'What could families and the local community do? – they are not trained'
14 'I don't know how to do evaluation'

clinical work concerned with planning, organising and supporting different aspects of an 'outreaching' District health care programme. Environmental health personnel may also be facing difficulties because they are highly trained in some areas (for example, maintenance of communal food markets) yet may find themselves doing a job where this skill is needed only very occasionally. The rest of the time they find that they are being asked to provide refuse or sewage services in a vast area with limited personnel and resources. Increasingly, in several countries competent and trained lay health administrators are becoming available. Their special skills can contribute greatly to the effective management of rural health services.

Districts vary from one country to another but from an organisational point of view many have similar features. In this book a 'model' for provision of health care is described which is already widely used in a number of African and Asian countries and is increasingly being adapted for use elsewhere. The principles are relevant everywhere. For example, there is increasing recognition in all countries that as much caring as possible should take place not in hospitals, but at the Primary Health Care level, within the community. For instance, in some rural parts of the United States traditional birth attendants do many deliveries, and physicians' assistants carry out many services in the absence of university-trained doctors. Increasingly, people's views about their services are being taken more into account.

The average District in mind has a population of between 200 000–500 000 though it could be as low as 100 000 in sparsely-populated countries or as high as one million. It covers varying areas from one country to another. There will be a District General Hospital (and possibly other hospitals) and a number of Health Centres and health posts, on the general principle of one Health Centre for every 100 000 population and one sub-centre for every 10 000 people.

All nations are now actively working towards the establishment of a viable primary health care programme. The District Health Team is expected to face this challenge and make the programme function effectively. The aim of this book is to look at the reality of translating plans into action and concepts into practice. Table 1.2 lists some of the problems discussed in the book.

Table 1.2 Do you experience these problems? (Tick)

Problems at the District level

No agreed plan for the District
No defined targets
Lack of adequate data to define District problems
Ignorance of activities taking place in the District
Lack of financial planning and a systematic way of allocating resources
Lack of interest, enthusiasm and understanding of what has to be done
Under-worked people
Over-worked people

Table 1.2   (*contd.*)

Problems in Hospitals

Wrong kinds of services are provided
Overwhelmed by demands
Divorced from community
No assessment of the community's health needs
Poor utilisation of resources, e.g. nurses' skills
No plans or targets
No clear policies or delegation
Hospital activities not integrated with Primary Health Care
Unrealistic aspirations
Poor financial control
No evaluation of hospital services

Problems at Health Centre level

Poorly trained staff
No regular in-service training
Lack of contact with villages
No support for community work
No procedures for routine activities
No defined targets
Lack of initiative
No community diagnosis
Over-strict demarcation of duties
Isolation from District officials and other workers
Unreliable deliveries of drugs and supplies; delayed payment of wages etc.
Poor morale
Lack of interest
Overspent budgets
Malpractices such as absenteeism, pilfering of drugs and misuse of vehicles
Unused and broken-down equipment
Badly-used buildings
Shortages of drugs, supplies and transport
Poor career structure and lack of job satisfaction
Problems at Health Centre level not recognised by District

Problems in the community

No services within reasonable reach
Mothers and babies die of preventable illness
Poor hygiene
Poor water supply
Lack of knowledge; ignorance
Shortage of leaders
Apathy, sense of futility
No priorities for tasks to be done
No links between health – education – agriculture – community development, i.e.
    no interdepartmental co-ordination

Table 1.2   (*contd.*)

Over-all problems

Lack of interest in management
Poor understanding of functions and roles, and of the health problems of the
    community
Misuse of resources
Lack of commitment and misplaced enthusiasm
Little contact with other departments like agriculture, education, social welfare,
    community development etc.
Constantly changing policies and priorities.

Problems such as these do not apply in all places and frequently progress is
made in very adverse conditions. Usually the best solutions to problems are
those which people work out for themselves and which best fit the local
situation. This book attempts to provide some guidance to help managers see
more clearly the nature of some of their problems and to suggest ideas which
may be helpful in resolving them.

WHY IS A NEW APPROACH TO HEALTH CARE NEEDED? HOW HAVE THE OLD APPROACHES FAILED?

Health services continue to grow yet health problems and health service inadequacies persist

Despite a heavy infusion of health care resources in many countries in the last
20 years, there is still a lack of health care in most areas. Table 1.3 shows data
from Ghana where there were huge increases in the number of health
personnel between 1960 and 1975, so that by 1975 the health worker:
population ratio looked quite good by any standard.

This table shows that since 1960 there have been remarkable increases in the
resources infused into the health services of Ghana, most notably in terms of
manpower and facilities. Yet despite this heavy infusion of resources, the
government recognised that by 1975 there had been little or no impact on the
health status of the population in general, and in particular on the 70 per cent
of the people who live in rural areas. Similar experience is not uncommon in
several countries.

Even with the increase in health manpower and hospital beds, clearly the
health problems and health service inadequacies are continuing. Table 1.4
shows the distribution of doctors in Ghana in 1975. Over a third were in the
capital city, Accra; another third were in the large towns and only the

Table 1.3 **The growth of health manpower and hospital beds, 1960-1975, Ghana**

Category of health personnel	1960	1975	Per cent increase 15 years	Population per health professional 1960	1975
Physicians	383	1 031	169%	17 564	9 625
Dental surgeons	19	60	216%	354 052	165 383
Nurses	1 554	6 153	296%	4 329	1 613
Midwives	130	4 932	3 694%	51 746	2 012
Hospital beds and cots	5 787	12 973	124%	1 162	765

Source: 1960 figures, The Health Services in Ghana, (1961), D. Brachott; 1975 figures, National Health Planning Unit, 1975 population estimate 9 923 000.

Table 1.4 **The problem of the distribution of doctors (Ghana, 1975)**

	% doctors	% population
Accra (the capital city)	34	7
Towns of more than 20 000 population	33	11
Places of less than 20 000 population	33	82

Source: Ghana Ministry of Health (1977), *Health Data book*, National Health Planning Unit. Population data from 1970 Census.

remaining third were to be found in the smaller communities, of under 20 000 people, where the majority of Ghana's population live. A similar pattern of distribution was likely to be found for midwives and environmental health workers. Table 1.5 gives the pattern of distribution of doctors in several other developing countries.

Apart from this obvious mismatch between health care provision and population distribution, another problem is apparent. Many deaths in the developing world still occur for reasons which could have been avoided through the provision of simple appropriate care. In many parts of the developing world up to 40 per cent of all children die before they reach school age (see table 1.6).

The tragedy is that, as in so many countries, the diseases could be prevented or controlled with Primary Health Care, by the use of immunisation, simple medications, environmental alterations and health education for the people. In the past ten years virtually no impact has been made on the prevalence of communicable diseases in many countries and some, like yaws and cholera,

Table 1.5   **Distribution of doctors between the capital and the
rest of the country, 1968**

Country	Population : Doctor Ratio		
	Nationwide	*Capital city*	*Rest of the country*
Kenya	10 000	672	25 600
Thailand	7 000	800	25 000
Guatemala	4 860	875	22 600
Jamaica	2 280	840	5 510
Pakistan	7 400	3 700	24 200
Philippines	3 900	1 500	10 000

Table 1.6   **Measures of ill-health in developing countries, 1970–75**

Region	Life expectancy at birth (years)	Infant mortality per 1000 live births	Mortality aged 1–4 per 1000	Crude birth rate per 1000
Tropical Africa	41	200	40	22
Northern Africa	52	150	26	15
Western South Asia	54	135	22	14
Middle South Asia	48	145	25	17
Eastern South Asia	51	120	18	15
Melanesia	48	150	–	17
East Asia	61	70	7	10
Caribbean	63	64	7	9
Tropical South America	61	100	10	9
Middle America	62	70	9	9

have increased dramatically. In addition, the maternal mortality rate remains
high, for example at over 40 per 10 000 deliveries in the rural areas of Ghana
and 42 per 10 000 births in India, which is several times more than the current
rate of less than 2 per 10 000 in Europe.

Not only are there high death rates due to preventable diseases but also there
are high rates of blindness, lameness and other forms of disability. Many of
these could be prevented or minimised with a Primary Health Care programme. A few countries have begun to measure the effects of high morbidity
rates on the national economy. For example, the National Health Planning
Unit in Ghana conducted a technical analysis of disease problems and their
impact on the level of health of the people. This is measured by estimating the
number of days of healthy life lost due to sickness, disability or death caused by
each sickness. The following are the sixteen major causes of sickness, disability
and death found (see table 1.7).

Table 1.7 Disease problems of Ghana ranked in order of impact on health status

Rank order	Disease classification	Days of healthy life lost*	Per cent of total
1	Malaria	58 427	15.4
2	Prematurity	34 432	9.1
3	Measles	23 033	6.1
4	Birth injury	22 612	6.0
5	Sickle-cell disease	21 797	5.9
6	Pneumonia, child	20 857	5.5
7	Kwashiorkor, marasmus	19 312	5.1
8	Dysentery & gastro-enteritis	17 022	4.5
9	Neonatal tetanus	14 047	3.7
10	Accidents (all kinds)	11 137	2.9
11	Tuberculosis	10 097	2.7
12	Cerebrovascular accidents (stroke)	8 915	2.4
13	Pneumonia, adult	8 743	2.3
14	Psychiatric disorders	8 542	2.3
15	Cancer	7 315	1.9
16	Pregnancy, complications of	6 005	1.6
Total of these 16 diseases		292 293	77.4%

* *Days of Healthy Life lost due to sickness, disability and death*: This is the number of days of healthy life estimated to be lost due to onset of disease (including the number of days in future years lost due to premature death or disability) in one year in population of 1000.

Example:
A man of 26 years develops tuberculosis and after 4 years sickness causing partial disability (25% disabled) he dies at age 30 years. He has lost 34 years of future expected life (plus one calculated year of 25% ($\frac{1}{4}$) disability over his 4 years with the disease; $4 \times \frac{1}{4} = 1$ year) i.e. 35 years of 365 days = 12 755 days of healthy life lost.
With the incidence of tuberculosis in Ghana being 2 per 1000 population per year, the average illness duration being 5 years and the average disability being 25%, as in the case above, in a population of 1000 two people will get tuberculosis disease each year. The case fatality rate is 30% (not everyone with tuberculosis dies, just 3 in 10 people). So the number of days of healthy life lost due to tuberculosis in a population of 1000 is 10 097 days per year.

Regional variations in mortality experience occur in all countries including the more developed countries. In the less developed countries, however, there is also the glaring urban/rural disparity so that infant and child mortality rates in rural areas are about a third higher than those for the cities. In recent years a further twist has been added to the question of disparities in the form of growing numbers of squatter settlements in most large cities. The mortality experience of the urban poor often exceeds that of the villages in spite of the relative proximity of the former to health care facilities. For example, in Manila the infant mortality rate is three times higher in the squatter areas than in the rest of the city, and in the *bustees* of New Delhi the over-all child mortality rate (0–5 years) reaches 440 per 1000 amongst certain groups.

Unequal distribution of health facilities resulting in disparities of health care is usually due to political and socio-economic factors. But disparities also indicate poor planning and management of health resources. Similar forces also operate at the Regional and District level as at the National level, leading to differences in health experience between communities. Some common symptoms of poor health management and planning are described in table 1.8.

Table 1.8 Some symptoms of poor health management

1 Adverse mortality and morbidity from preventable illness. High infant mortality. Major differences in mortality rates and life expectancy between communities.

2 Health facilities geographically inaccessible on account of urban bias, and rural inadequacy. In some countries up to 85% of the population in rural areas have no access to any form of modern health care.

3 People cannot afford to pay for health services, or the costs of time away from work, transport, etc.

4 Curative care is emphasised to the neglect of prevention and early treatment. Institutional care is the common practice rather than care provided near the home within the community.

5 More money is spent on hospitals than on simple Primary Health Care facilities, with up to 80% of health spending being on 'Western' type hospital care.

6 The wrong kinds of health workers are trained, with an emphasis on training highly qualified doctors and specialists instead of auxiliaries with basic skills.

7 Health services are often imposed from above and do not always have the support of local communities.

8 The Health Care provided is inappropriate for the main health needs. Infections, parasitic and respiratory diseases, are often widespread and have relatively simple preventive solutions if implemented on a wide scale, but health resources are often devoted mainly to curative services.

9 Demographic pressures are increasing with disproportionate increases in numbers of babies and children. This causes demands for maternal and child health services which are neglected in favour of fashionable intensive care.

10 Severe economic problems force governments and planners to impose drastic cuts so that essential drugs and supplies become scarce with periodic shortages.

11 Widespread poverty causes environmental problems, shortage of water and natural resources.

12 Breakdowns in conventional medical systems where they exist, e.g., overcrowding of facilities, misuse of technical equipment, shortages of supplies, unresponsiveness to chronic diseases and handicap.

13 Isolation and weak support of existing primary health care services and workers, leading to a discrediting of the contribution they can make.

14 Difficulties in implementing individual 'vertical' health programmes on a massive scale (e.g., malaria prevention, leprosy control, programmes for eye diseases) and maintaining their effectiveness on a permanent basis.

15 More interest amongst some health planners in detailed research and lengthy reports than in contact with local people and implementation of appropriate programmes.

16 Unwillingness of the health establishment to involve existing human resources in the community for extending health coverage.

Why no improvement in health?

The data presented in the preceding paragraphs indicate that despite a very great increase in the resources devoted to the health sector in the last ten years, there has been little improvement in over-all health status and health service provision for the majority of people. One basic reason for this seems to be that the health services have been doing the wrong things because of misplaced priorities. This is as true at the District level as at the National level. The existing health service system funnels resources towards the minority of populations having access to hospital-based services catering largely for specialised health problems (see figure 1.1).

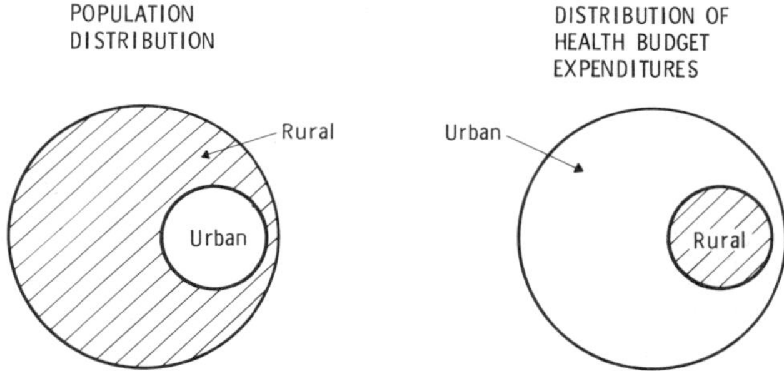

Figure 1.1   Undesirable distribution of health budget expenditures

In many countries, for understandable but self-defeating reasons, hospital-based curative services requiring highly trained personnel and expensive equipment have received the greatest amount of attention and have commanded the bulk of resources (up to 80 per cent) set aside for health care by the government. This has created a paradoxical situation. Because of inadequate public health and Primary Health Care services, patients with preventable conditions have over-loaded the hospital services so that tertiary care facilities are being used for primary care. On the other hand, overcrowding in hospitals leads to greater demand for more hospitals. As more resources are put into the construction and equipping of hospitals and the training of sophisticated health workers required for their operation, even less resources become available to develop the Primary Health Care system (see figure 1.2).

For most preventable conditions (parasitic diseases, nutritional disorders, common infections, illnesses of childhood, etc.) the elaborate hospital care required after the disease is established is not only expensive, but is also only partially effective, thus compounding the consequences of this inappropriate allocation of resources. It is an unfortunate paradox that the *demand* for services occurs only after illness becomes evident: while the *need* for services is long before illness occurs.

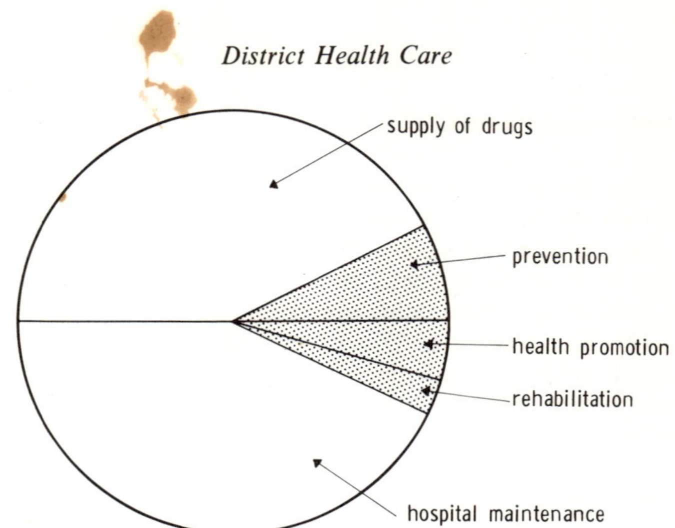

Figure 1.2   Unbalanced health budget allocations

The people, their elders, leaders and chiefs, and therefore the political decision-makers often perceive the basic issues of health care in terms of hospitals and doctors. This view is often reinforced by doctors themselves who have been trained in the sophisticated, intellectually intriguing disciplines of diagnosis and therapy of individually ill people. Their attention is focused on the sick who seek their help. But the need is to maintain the health of *those who are not yet ill*.

This situation is strikingly illustrated in figure 1.3 describing the health care dilemma of the average developing country, taking Ghana as an example. It shows how the financial resources of the nation are being allocated in reverse proportion to the number of people in need!

Five main reasons have been identified as the cause of this situation in which many countries, developing and developed alike, find themselves. These are:

(1) Focus on the construction of facilities rather than the provision of services.
(2) Over-sophisticated training which takes place largely inside hospitals with emphasis on specialised hospital-based services rather than preventive and promotive services.
(3) Poor and unequitable deployment of health staff.
(4) A 'top-down' health care delivery system with a noticeable lack of co-ordination with other sectors (social welfare and community development, water and sewerage, education, agriculture, etc.) and little or no community involvement.
(5) Unbalanced health budget allocations.

The present health care system of many countries can be likened to a pyramid with the Teaching or District Hospital at the top, as the case may be,

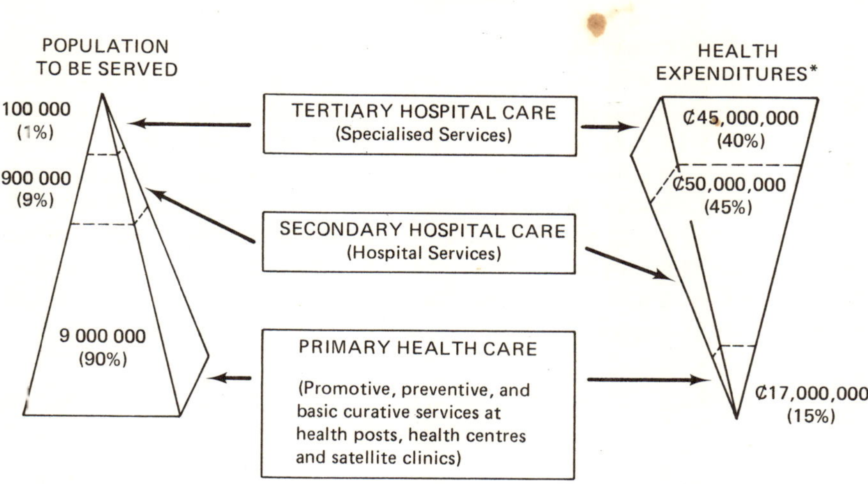

*Approximations based on 1975/76 estimates
₡ = Cedi, the currency in Ghana

Figure 1.3   The health care dilemma in Ghana. (The distribution of funds and personnel for primary health care compared to costly hospital-based care is in inverse proportion to the numbers of people that need to be reached. The Health Care Pyramid is upside down!)

Source: Primary Health Care Strategy for Ghana, National Health Planning Unit, 1979.

and a network of health posts and dressing stations at the bottom. This is a system based on health units (that is, structural facilities). It focuses attention on 'bricks and mortar' rather than on health services. This emphasis on structural facilities creates false 'needs' among the people for more facilities. Good health becomes synonymous with the provision of a doctor and a hospital rather than the enjoyment of a disease-free environment.

Under these conditions, each community without a health post believes it should have one for reasons of prestige; each community with a health post wants to expand it into a Health Centre; and each community with a Health Centre sees a 'need' to add a surgical theatre and ward and bring a surgeon to town. The pressure continues upward to Regional and National levels with its attendant burgeoning demands for financial and manpower resources. This upward pressure absorbs all available resources and leaves an ever-increasing vacuum at the bottom of the pyramid where the real health needs of the nation lie.

The approach adopted in many countries up until the 1960s and 1970s was based on systems of health care in use in Western developed countries, forgetting that the main strength of the health system (for example, in Britain) lay in the grass-roots viz. the general practitioner and the health visitor.

Instead, the systems created in many developing countries relied heavily on skilled manpower and on a curative approach to disease through the use of drugs, surgical and other invasive techniques. But in such a system care was available only to small numbers of the population, mainly those with the ability to pay and with easy access to hospitals, trained staff, and other facilities situated mainly in the cities and urban areas. This approach to health care has had only a modest impact on the health of the vast majority of the population in most developing countries. Though not present in all countries, many of the symptoms of poor health management shown in table 1.8 and figure 1.4 are frequently found.

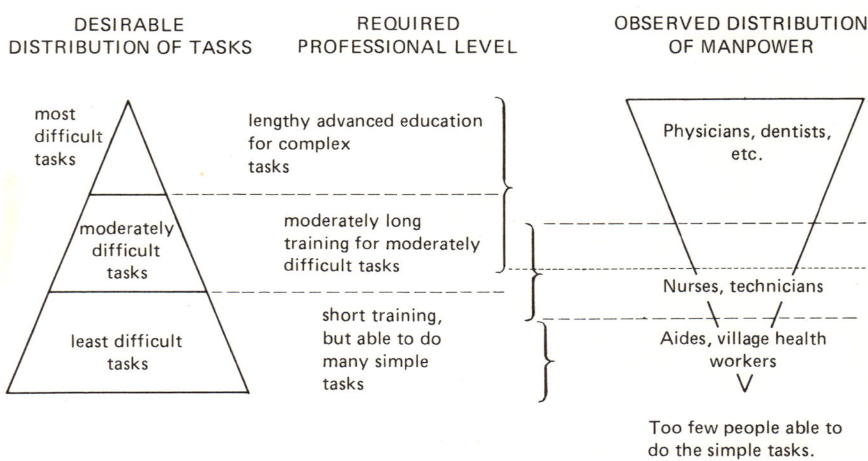

Figure 1.4   Why no improvement in health? Poor deployment of health staff

Extra problems exacerbating the difficulties of health care planning

Two additional interrelated factors compound the problems of misplaced priorities:

(1) The rapid population growth and its impact on the per capita expenditure available for health and development.
(2) Raging inflation together with the devaluation of many local currencies.

The crude birth rate in many countries persists at a level of 45 to 55 per 1000 population. At the present estimated growth rate of over 3 per cent per year, the population of many countries will double in about 20 years. This exponential growth in population means that each year more and more people must share the 'national cake' of the health services. The portion available to each person is shrinking steadily (see figure 1.5).

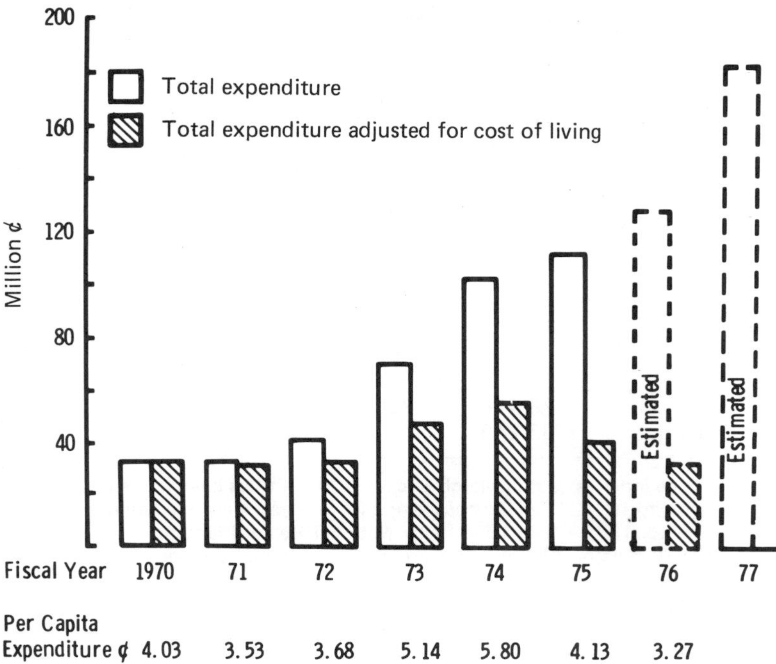

Figure 1.5   Ghana Ministry of Health expenditure adjusted for cost of living and population growth 1971–1977

Even when governments can increase health expenditure the amount of goods and services the money will buy may still become smaller and smaller if the increased expenditure does not keep up with inflation. Table 1.9 and figure 1.5 illustrate this problem in the case of Ghana. In Iraq the increase in health manpower between 1956 and 1975 has been between 177 and 334 per cent, depending upon the category of the health worker. During this period health expenditure increased by 226 per cent for a population which increased by 227 per cent. But because of the inflation which can be estimated at 250 per cent between 1956 and 1975, the health expenditure in real terms actually declined. Thus the government's ability to finance services is decreasing in many countries and the traditional concept of building a network of hospitals, Health Centres and health posts needs to be reviewed. In any case the priority disease problems do not merit continuation of such a policy.

Clearly something different is needed. But as if these facts were not enough, the present shortages of food and simple necessities of life in many countries, the increasing poverty among some nations and the obvious leap in malnutrition in many young children in some countries in the last five years, shows that poverty-caused and poverty-related health problems need urgent and increasing attention. This explains the reason why the District Health

Table 1.9 **Ministry of Health expenditures – Ghana (adjusted for cost of living and population growth 1971 – 1977)**

Fiscal Year	Total expend. (¢ 000)	Consumer price index*	Total expend. adjusted for cost of living	Per capita expend. adjusted**
1970–71	34 505	197.3	34 505	¢ 4.03
1971–72	34 026	216.4	31 023	3.51
1972–73	41 965	246.6	33 575	3.68
1973–74	71 223	290.9	48 306	5.14
1974–75	103 279	362.1	56 274	5.80
1975–76	112 095	534.0	41 416	4.13
1976–77 (budget)	128 414	750.0 (est.)	33 781	3.27
1977–78 (budget)	183 745	(not available)		

* Consumer price index based on March 1963 = 100. This has been adjusted to equate all years in this table to 1970–71 as the base year. Figures shown are average of the two years listed. Estimates for 1975–6 and 1976–7 by National Health Planning Unit.
** Based on 1970 census of 8 559 000 increased at an annual average rate of 3.2% for the subsequent years.

Source: Ministry of Finance. Central Bureau of Statistics. Ghana Census, 1970.

Teams should not expect to see real improvement in District health budgets in the foreseeable future.

A NEW APPROACH TO HEALTH CARE AND ITS MANAGEMENT REQUIREMENTS

The origins of the new approach

In the light of these problems concerning the existing health care system, many countries are now evolving more effective ways of improving health in their communities. Some of the significant developments are summarised in table 1.10.

Features of Primary Health Care

A number of countries are adopting new approaches to health care. There are two major objectives, (1) to design health services which can reach the majority of the people, and (2) to prevent and treat the preventable disease problems which are presently responsible for much ill health (morbidity as well as disability) and mortality. Both these objectives are to be achieved through community involvement and participation which require a high level of awareness.

The principal means of implementing this approach is through a Primary Health Care system aimed at reducing the rates of mortality and morbidity caused by conditions for which prevention, easy treatment and control exist. Prominent among these causes in many countries are communicable diseases, nutritional deficiencies and manageable complications of pregnancy. Priority for health improvement is then determined by which procedures can produce the greatest reduction in the unnecessary burden of sickness, disability and death, at the least cost. Most of the health improvement procedures that will have the greatest impact are simple tasks that can be carried out by people without sophisticated training using simple equipment, provided there are satisfactory organisational arrangements for the needed support and supervision. This new approach to health care provision is seen as part of the national effort in social and economic development with community involvement at each level and support from health centres and hospitals. Together they make up the system for primary health care.

However, there is no 'right' or 'wrong' way of providing primary health care in a country, or even to all regions of a single country. Countries and communities vary in terms of size, geography, climate, population, communications, level of political, economic and social development, health needs and resources, and local leadership. Systems of providing health care need to be evolved which meet each locality's circumstances and problems. It is important also that a country feels confident that it has developed a system which meets its own needs, and which, because it has been developed by its own people, has the commitment and determination of its people to make it work. But there are certain features of primary health services which are increasingly being widely adopted. These are shown in table 1.11.

Management requirements for successful Primary Health Care

The success of a Primary Health Care system depends on a number of factors, in particular National and local commitment, National strategy to provide guidelines, a local District plan building on local experience, a District Health Team as part of a multi-level structure with clearly defined roles which recognise the different tasks in hospital and community, and local community involvement. The following requirements for success in setting up a District programme for Primary Health Care can be identified:

(1) *Awareness* among health workers, health planners and lay people of basic health problems.

**Table 1.10 Significant new developments to solve the problems
in existing health care provision**

1   A commitment on the part of a number of governments to give priority to primary health care for disadvantaged groups.

2   Recognition that many diseases widespread in the population lend themselves to relatively simple non-medical solutions, e.g., improvements in water supply, hygiene, nutrition, etc.

3   Recognition of the social nature of much ill-health like the lack of services for the rural areas and for the urban poor which calls for a sociological and political rather than medical approach.

4   Recognition of community development, whereby the development of a community in all its aspects, family welfare, farming, income-earning activities, social functioning, child-rearing, community action, etc., is seen as having a vital part to play in improving not only health, but other aspects of development.

5   Greater awareness of the need for co-operation between agencies, e.g., education, agriculture, health, to ensure a sharing of resources and a co-ordinated approach to problems.

6   Development of 'Bottom-up' as opposed to 'Top-down' planning, i.e., taking the needs, resources and opportunities in local communities as the starting point for planning health services, as opposed to planning on the basis solely of needs and policies as seen at the national level.

7   Increasing awareness amongst ordinary people of their lack of health care and growing demands for something to be done about it.

8   Because of difficulties in implementing individual 'vertical' health programmes over unduly long periods (e.g., malaria, leprosy) a recognition of the need for 'general care' rather than 'specialist cure' programmes.

9   Recognition of the value of 'screening' techniques for large numbers especially among the vulnerable groups like children and pregnant and lactating women in the population to detect signs of disease at an early stage.

10 Recognition that with alternative methods of health care delivery, considerable improvements in people's health can be made at relatively low cost.

11 Recognition of non-financial resources which are often present in rural communities, e.g., social cohesion, traditional skills, enthusiasm when encouraged and motivated.

12 Growth of experience from different countries – e.g., of 'barefoot doctors' in China; health services 'where there is no doctor', in Mexico; planned health services at low cost in Tanzania.

13 Renewed interest by professionals in traditional cures and herbal medicines, in many parts of the world – in Africa, Asia, North America, China.

14 Application of 'appropriate technology' to health care, e.g., coloured strip for measuring arm circumference, rehydration spoons, simple weighing machines, low cost hand pumps for water supply etc.

15 Changes in medical training with a better understanding of psychological and social factors affecting health, and an appreciation of the need to train larger numbers of health workers with more appropriate skills.

16 Recognition of the enormous contribution which can be made to the provision of health care by groups hitherto under-utilised in the community, e.g., women, nurses, children.

Table 1.11   **Features of primary health care increasingly being adopted**

1   *Focus on the community*
  1.1   Emphasis on health care at the village or community level
  1.2   Use of local community workers at the first level of health care, drawn from and supported by the community
  1.3   Involvement of the community in the planning and running of their own health services
  1.4   Use of traditional methods and resources, e.g., the traditional birth attendant.

2   *Emphasis on hygiene and prevention of disease*
  2.1   Promotion of mother and child health services including immunisation and nutrition
  2.2   Environmental and public health given equal stress as curative care
  2.3   Emphasis on health education.

3   *Planning for services relevant to local needs*
  3.1   Identification of major health problems and adoption of specific programmes to combat them
  3.2   Regular evaluation to ensure continual improvement of health programme
  3.3   Strategies for improving coverage and for developing low-cost technology, e.g., limited drug formularies, low-cost waste disposal systems etc.
  3.4   Integration of health with other aspects of development, e.g., agriculture, education, community development and so on.

4   *Organisation of services to improve utilisation and quality of care*
  4.1   Provision of basic health care facilities within walking distance for the majority of the population
  4.2   A hierarchy of levels of health care comprising 3 key elements: local community; Health Centre/sub-centre complex; District Hospital
  4.3   Different levels of District health facilities becoming supportive of each other and of community-based health activities

5   *Training based on locally assessed needs*
  5.1   Health workers at each hierarchy of care trained in preventive and environmental health as well as to diagnose and treat a limited number of common illnesses, less common diseases not included in the training being referred to the next higher level of care
  5.2   Continuing education to improve skills at all levels of care

(2) *Commitment* to improve the health of the population, both for its own sake and as a foundation for economic and social development. This is as true at the district level as at the national level. This commitment needs to be expressed throughout the health system as a commitment to *Primary Health Care*. A balance needs to be maintained between primary and secondary care, and this may mean drastic and determined action where hospitals have expanded disproportionately. This entails a commitment to equitable *financing* and shifting of expenditure from the

tertiary level to the primary care level. Commitment is also needed amongst medical, nursing and other professional staff. Much is being done in some medical schools to select and train doctors to work in Primary Health Care where the attitudes, skills and conditions of work are very different from those appropriate to hospitals or private urban practice. A positive commitment to primary health care is even more important at higher ministerial levels where policies are made and resources allocated for health care.

(3) The national commitment ideally finds expression in a *National Strategy*. Many countries have produced a National Health Plan which sets out a broad strategy and takes into account those factors which are best planned for nationally, for example:

manpower planning to establish in broad terms the numbers and roles of health workers needed;

training programmes, for example, medical assistants, public health nurses, environmental health workers;

'vertical' health programmes, for example, malaria eradication;

simple and appropriate agreements on drug formularies and purchasing of drugs;

design of effective health education material.

Within the framework of such a National Plan, effective District Plans need to be produced and attention given to the demanding task of implementing the plan.

(4) It is unlikely that a District Health Team will set about its task completely from scratch. Every society in order to survive has developed its own ways of coping with disease, and maintaining a state of health amongst its population. This will include feeding habits, housing arrangements, practices affecting pregnancy, child-rearing, care of old people, means of coping with disease, accidents and tragedy. Where traditional practices are effective they need to be maintained and encouraged. Health problems often arise because traditional practices, for example, birth-spacing, breast feeding, balanced diets, have been neglected in the face of 'modern developments' associated with such things as higher cash income, increased mobility, 'status' foods like carbonated drinks, powdered milk, packaged weaning foods etc. Beneficial practices and traditional health resources need to be encouraged and incorporated into the district health programme.

Some health programmes may already exist like Country Health Programmes organised on a national basis; health-related programmes run by other agencies, for example, agriculture, community development, religious bodies, various forms of private medicine (doctors in private practice, retail chemists, services provided by employers); hospitals which provide primary health care. The task of a local management team is to identify what is already taking place, support and develop it and knit it into whatever new activities and services may be planned.

The greatest challenge is how to make the people feel that the health system is 'theirs'; that they own it, take pride in it, and support it, because it meets their needs and fits in with local traditions.

(5) *Community involvement*. The greatest resource available is likely to be the community itself and it can be the foundation on which the whole health system is built. Over the past 30 years many countries have made large investments to build up the industrial and commercial base of economic development in the belief that this would lead to the building up of an educated élite and an urban middle class and that consequent economic benefits would 'trickle down' to all sections of the community and act as a spur to development amongst the mass of the rural poor. This theory is now being questioned. What this approach to development ignored was that the greatest potential asset of any country lies in its own people's resourcefulness and their will to work for the improvement of their living conditions. To work well people need to be healthy, and this means that health services have a crucial part to play in the over-all development programme.

Moreover, health programmes can themselves be a 'trigger' for further development, by mobilising the resources and capabilities of communities to fulfil their own aspirations. Guidance and assistance can be welcomed by rural communities to build their own health services if it is genuinely offered in practical ways which the local population feel are appropriate. The skills and understanding of how to work *with* communities in this way are fundamental to successful primary health care. (After all, getting things done with people is what management is all about.) The understanding is rooted in the academic disciplines of psychology, sociology, communication, anthropology and other human sciences which are being given increased attention in the training of health workers, supplemented by field work to understand community interactions in a local population and its ways of living. But the attitude is basically a personal one in which health workers say 'We have certain medical skills, and know-how about how people can keep themselves healthy, but it is the community who best knows how this knowledge can be applied. Therefore we need to get to know the community, be trusted by the people in it, and work *with* local people to provide the services they need'. Furthermore, involving the communities in the identification of their needs, planning health programmes, implementing and evaluating them, raises their level of awareness of their health and other problems and commits them to doing something about their problems.

(6) The *District Health Team* (DHT) is a key element in the thinking behind this book. A District Medical Officer (DMO) does not work in isolation.

Primary Health Care is a comprehensive system of care, prevention, treatment, community development, management and organisation. Yet few doctors possess all the skills and knowledge required, nor have control over all the health workers and resources in the District.

At the district level there may be such people as:

Medical assistants, and other auxiliary workers.

A senior public health nurse with responsibility for midwives, public health nurses and community nurses.

A senior environmental health officer responsible for environmental health with a staff of public health inspectors, sanitarians, assistants, etc.

A senior nutrition worker, responsible for monitoring the nutrition extension work at the health institutions and in the community.

A Health Education Officer.

Administrators/Finance Officers/Supplies staff with responsibilities for primary health care.

Together such people can work as a team with one or more persons designated as managers. However, it should be recognised that management of primary health care is a different management task from that of a hospital (see table 1.12).

Together such people can work as a team with one District Medical Officer accepting a joint responsibility for Primary Health Care. In addition such people as Community Development Officers, Education officials, Agriculture and Veterinary officers, community leaders, may work closely with a District Health Team. But it is the small 'core' DHT which is the 'nerve centre' and powerhouse for overseeing the work of the District and carrying out the functions of planning, developing, maintaining and evaluating services; supporting, building and developing staff and systems of work; and maintaining links between the local situation and government, regional and other agencies. Whilst having a joint responsibility for the district as a whole, each team member retains responsibility for his/her own specialised activities. The 'team' approach provides an opportunity for better joint decisions; consideration of a wider range of ideas and suggestions; support from members of the team to one another; unity, so that key staff and 'managers' in the district speak with a common voice; common policies agreed by all; continuity, whereby the team continues even if one person is absent; and a recognised means of settling differences and problems between people who work together.

Working relationships may need to be clarified where there is a District Hospital in the same District. A management team may be involved in running the hospital, for example, a Medical Director, Matron and Hospital Secretary, and there may also be some common membership between the Hospital Management Team and the District

Table 1.12 Management of primary health care is a different kind of management task from that of the hospital

Hospital	*Health Centre has both features*	*Primary Health Care*
Complex systems		Relatively simple system
High technology		Low technology
High capital investment		Low capital investment
High technical skill in small numbers of trained staff		More of low technical skill – widely distributed
Changing patient population – relatively shallow personal relationships		Stable community population – deeper personal relationships
Professionals do things to patients (passive patient)		Health workers do things *with* mothers, families (active client involvement)
High degree of specialisation – specialist doctors, nurses, technicians		Health workers are multi-purpose and do many tasks – diagnosis, treatment, clerking, social work, nursing
Short-term visible results, individual patients get better		Long term results, not always visible – the health of the community improves over a period of time
Disease centred – responds to disease demands presented to it		'Health' centred – identifies total community health *needs* and acts on them.
Prestigious. Patients and staff want to come to it		Low-key, mundane – some people want to get away from it
Comparatively rich		Poor – financially and educationally
Calls for high order administrative procedural skills (tendency to strict, autocratic management, e.g., in operating theatre)		Calls for high order personal and social skills and common-sense and adaptability. Needs open, encouraging, participative management style
'Alien' system introduced from outside – an urban institution		Integrated and woven into the fabric of the community
Grows from external resources		Grows from internal resources
Highly structured hierarchical organisation		Individuals and small groups work on their own and often in isolation
Creates its own dynamism		Dynamism must be maintained

Health Team. Where this is so, the functions and scope of each team will need to be defined clearly.

There can be special problems in relating the work of primary health care to that of a hospital. A hospital's main function is to provide secondary care (or tertiary care). The nature of primary and secondary care is essentially different, and table 1.12 sets out some of the major differences managers may need to bear in mind.

Where manpower and other constraints do not permit, Health Teams can be set up to manage District health services.

(7) *A multi-level structure.* Remarkably similar structures are being developed in a number of countries in East and West Africa, Asia, and elsewhere. A basic 3–4-level system operates as follows:

Level A – Village or small community, serving a population of about 500–1000. The community is involved through a village health committee and village health workers working in association with traditional birth attendants and local healers. Services provided are mainly in the fields of prevention, hygiene and sanitation, first aid, simple diagnosis and treatment, antenatal and postnatal care, child care and control of communicable diseases.

Level B$_1$ – A sub-centre or health post serving a population of 5000–10 000, staffed by 2 to 3 paid workers, for example, rural medical and nursing aide, midwifery aides, and so on. It provides diagnostic and outpatient service, holding beds for acutely ill patients, antenatal and under-fives' clinics and midwifery services. Some countries have only a midwifery centre at Level B, whilst in others Levels B$_1$ and B$_2$ are combined for administrative reasons.

Level B$_2$ – Health Centre serving a number of sub-centres (in practice, any number from 5 to 20) and a population of about 50 000–100 000, staffed by a small number of paid workers, for example, a medical assistant, public health nurse/midwife, environmental health worker/sanitarian. The health centre provides clinic, diagnostic and treatment services for patients referred by village health workers and sub-centres. It also supports village health workers to ensure that as much work as possible is done at the village level.

Level C – The District level serving a population of between 200 000–500 000. A District Health Team is responsible for planning, administration and support of Health Centres, health posts and village health workers throughout the District, and providing help to patients and problems referred to them from Health Centres. Services may also be provided in a District Hospital or through a District Health facility in which more advanced services and treatments are provided than are possible in Health Centres. District mobile teams may provide services throughout the District and support the work of Health Centres.

Beyond the District level there is the National level (Ministry of Health) and in large countries an intermediate Provincial or Regional level. Variations of the basic 'multi-level' approach depend on geography, population, resources available, and so on, but it is important to incorporate the main principles of the approach in any local arrangement (see table 1.13).

(8) *Clearly understood roles*. Those who work within a Primary Health Care system must have a clear idea of what they are doing and trying to

Table 1.13 Principles in establishing a multi-level structure

(a) The village and local community as the foundation for all health services.

(b) Services provided at as local a level as possible, by health workers trained to make the greatest impact on the most common health problems of their locality.

(c) Support from more distant levels (C and B) to local levels (B and A) in the form of training, encouragement, supplies, etc.

(d) More distant levels deal *only* with the relatively few cases and problems which cannot be dealt with at local levels.

(e) Concentration of technical expertise at District level but readily available and constantly supportive for use throughout the District.

(f) A co-ordinated multi-disciplinary and multi-activity approach. Thus at village (local community) level, the village health committee (or in some cases village development committee) and village health workers are concerned with prevention, care, environmental health and simple treatments; at sub-centre and Health Centre level each worker has his or her special function, but with a good deal of inter-changeability; and at District level, the District Health Team of specialist professionals work together to plan and support a co-ordinated approach to the health needs of the District as a whole.

(g) Hospitals where they exist, are incorporated into the health care system of the District as a whole rather than operating as separate institutions.

achieve. A number of quite distinct roles can be identified; for example

> Village health worker
>
> Traditional birth attendant
>
> Health Centre Superintendent who may be a doctor as in India, an auxiliary as in Tanzania, or a trained nurse as in Ghana.
>
> District Medical Officer
>
> District Co-ordinator of Mother and Child Health (MCH)

These roles are quite specific to Primary Health Care and need to be related to the needs and requirements of the particular local situation. Individuals holding these roles may have had formal training (for example, as a nurse or a doctor) but that training may not be sufficient in itself and will need supplementing and developing. Over a period of time conditions also change, and roles need to be flexible enough to adapt. Outlines are given of the main functions of a Primary Health Worker (see table 1.14) and of the managerial role of doctors in community medicine in developing countries (see table 1.15). Such roles would need to be understood by the individuals who hold them and by their supervisors, but also by other professionals, colleagues and the community with whom they relate so as to avoid unrealistic expectations.

(9) *Clearly defined systems.* Within this structure there are a number of *systems* which need to function well if good health care is to be provided. To use the analogy of the body, the 4-level structure provides the skeleton or anatomy of the District, but a number of systems also need

Table 1.14 **The primary health worker (PHW) profile**

PHW Organisational Relationships
The PHW is responsible both to the local community and to a supervisor appointed by the national health services.
The PHW follows the instructions given by a supervisor and will work with him or her as a member of a team.

Duties of the PHW:
1 Cares for the health of the members of his community and promotes community hygiene.
2 Gives care and advice during illness and arranges for referral if necessary.
3 Refers patients to the nearest Health Centre or hospital if they cannot be treated by him locally. The PHW should therefore confine care and treatment to those cases, conditions and situations for which he is adequately trained.
4 Where necessary, visits homes and gives advice on how to prevent disease and develop good habits of hygiene.
5 Makes regular reports to the local authorities on the health of the people and on the conditions of hygiene in the community. Gets the local authorities and the people to give him the help and support he needs for his work.
6 Keeps in regular contact with his supervisor so as to be able to give of his best in his work and to obtain the equipment and supplies he needs.
7 Promotes community development activities and plays an active part in them. This assumes that the PHW:
   (a) is available to respond to any emergency calls
   (b) acts in all circumstances with commonsense and in awareness of his or her limitations and of his or her responsibilities
   (c) does not leave the community without first informing the local authorities (village development and/or health committee)
   (d) takes part in the periods of training organised by the health service
   (e) motivates parents and families to make use of available health services e.g. MCH clinics.
The PHW may spend some time with other social/developmental workers involved in improving agricultural practices, storage of food, water supply, home economics, etc. The PHW needs to know about development opportunities in the district and must keep the community properly informed.

(Adapted from 'The Primary Health Worker Working Guide' pp. 3–5, WHO 1977).

to work effectively and in harmony with one another. Such systems include:

Systems for diagnosis, referral, treatment and care of patients.

Systems for antenatal, postnatal and child care.

Systems for identifying and tackling the community's major health problems, for example, communicable diseases.

Transport and communication systems.

Systems to do with management of staff, for example, recruitment, training.

Systems for the procurement and distribution of drugs, equipment and other supplies.

Table 1.15 **Analysis of the managerial role of doctors in community medicine in developing countries**

Content of work

1	*Technical skills*	e.g. Diagnosis and Treatment of: (a) Individuals (b) Communities
2	*Teaching*	i.e. Giving other people the knowledge and skills to perform competently
3	*Management of resources*	Management of finance, e.g., general budgeting and financial control. Personnel management, e.g., arrangement of clinic sessions Disposition of Vehicles Allocating and delegating work to others
4	*Data gathering*	e.g. Demographic profile of the district; epidemiological characteristics and health statistics.
5	*Planning*	Thinking and planning ahead to determine what should be done in the future.
6	*Innovation and development*	i.e. Introducing new approaches and development to achieve better results e.g. Encouraging, supporting the work of others. Giving a sense of direction.
7	*Community mobilisation*	e.g. Involving the community on the day-to-day level in planning implementation and evaluation of health programmes.
8	*Minor administrative matters*	
9	*Dealing with crises*	

FURTHER READING

Ebrahim, G. J. A model of integrated community health care in a rural area. *Trop. and Geog. Med.* (1976) **28**: Supplement.

Walt, G. and Vaughan, P. *An introduction to the primary health care approach in developing countries.* Ross Institute Publication No. 13. 1981.

World Health Organization. *Primary Health Care.* WHO 'Health for All' Series No. 1, Geneva, 1978.

2 Finding Out About Health Needs in the District

When therefore a physician comes to a district previously unknown, its situation and its aspect to the winds must be considered. This is of the greatest importance and the effect of each season of the year must be studied. Similarly the nature of the water supply must be considered; then the soil, whether it be bare and waterless or thickly covered with vegetation. Is the area hollow and stifling or exposed and cold. Lastly consider the life of the inhabitants themselves; are they heavy drinkers and eaters and consequently unable to withstand fatigue or, being fond of work and exercise eat wisely and drink sparely?

Hippocrates: *Airs, Waters, Places*

The five key questions in community diagnosis of sickness are raised in this quotation. Who becomes sick? Where? When? With what? and Why? The same five questions are also applied to identifying health care resources; Who is providing care? What? Where? When? And we need to ask Why? as well for there are many different reasons why a particular pattern of health service develops. In order to decide what actions are needed in a district these two sets of five questions need to be asked to identify the specific problems and the resources available to deal with them.

In addition, community diagnosis needs also to describe community factors. It needs to describe the pattern of disease not just in terms of types of disease but also in terms of causation, for example, infectious agents and their prevalence, food production, life-style, beliefs and attitudes, and so on. It is not enough simply to say that people do not cultivate enough food. Answers are also needed to questions such as 'Why aren't people cultivating enough food crops?' 'Is the soil unsuitable?' 'Is there a shortage of land for some people?' 'Is there more scope for change within the community in relation to some things, for example, "soft points" compared with other aspects which are far less likely to change, that is, "hard points"?'

WHO? WHAT? WHERE? WHEN? WHY? IN ILL HEALTH

Which age groups contain most people and which age group is increasing fastest?

The age structure of the population in a District is the first indicator of what the pattern of health problems is likely to be. In many developing countries children under five make up about 20 per cent of the population and women and children together often account for as many as 65 per cent of the people. Older people, over 65, are also a rapidly increasing age group all over the world. The precise situation in a District can be obtained from census data corrected for the annual growth rate since the census was taken. In one district in Ghana, Ashanti-Akim, it was found that women of child-bearing age and children under 15 made up 65 per cent of the population (see table 2.1). Such a pattern of population is typical of most developing countries and is the result of a high birth rate coupled with low life expectancy.

Table 2.1 Population of the district from census data (1970) (corrected, allowing for 3% growth rate per annum) Ashanti-Akim District Profile, 1979

Population of district	156 000	
Total under 5	29 299	(19%)
Total under age 15	78 000	(50%)
Women of child-bearing age	23 217	(15%)
Total Women of child-bearing age and children under 15	101 217	(65%)

Who gets sick? Who dies?

The heavy burden of ill health borne by children can often be seen from the high proportion of child deaths amongst the top ten causes of deaths occurring in a District Hospital. Nearly a quarter of hospital deaths may be children. For every child that dies there is a bereaved family in need of emotional and social support. Although maternal deaths may thankfully be less frequent, when a mother dies several children may suffer and a household may lose a major contributor to its labour force.

Tables 2.2 and 2.3 give the most common causes of death in hospitals in Ghana and in Tanzania. In the case of the former, up to one in four deaths were in children and in the case of the latter, one in three deaths occurred in children. Disease problems often occur more frequently in certain age-groups, and in certain families, as well as in those who have been frequently ill before. Malnourished children are far more likely to fall ill, develop serious illness and

Table 2.2   **Top ten causes of death in one year – Agogo District Hospital, Ashanti-Akim District Profile, 1979 (N = 5056 admissions)**

	% of total
Premature and neonatal	13.9
Kwashiorkor malnutrition	10.0
Heart disease	8.9
Liver disease	7.9
Pulmonary disease	6.7
Malaria	6.3
Septicaemia	6.2
Intestinal disease	6.1
Tuberculosis	5.4
Measles	4.6

Table 2.3   **Most common causes of deaths in hospitals, Tanzania 1972**

	% of Total
Pneumonia	15.6
Diarrhoeal disease	9.6
Malaria	4.4
Tuberculosis	4.7
Diseases of the heart	4.5
Meningitis	0.9
Defective nutrition	7.1
Anaemia	4.8
Conditions of early infancy	6.9
Measles	10.5
Tetanus	4.6

succumb to it compared to children who are well nourished. Malnourished children under the age of five are particularly prone to diarrhoea. In a recent survey of Kwale District in Kenya (population 267 000) diarrhoea was the main complaint for which children were brought to its 121 health units and occurred in 15 per cent of 235 children under the age of five years. Diarrhoea did not feature at all as a major complaint in 148 children aged 5 to 15, nor in 200 adults.

Who needs maternity care?

The size of the need for maternity care in the District is partly indicated by the number of births. This figure can be obtained by using the National crude birth rate and the District population to calculate the District births expected. This can be compared with the District total of registered births. Often there are discrepancies between these numbers since in many countries few births are registered.

Table 2.4 Number of births expected and found registered (1978) Ashanti-Akim district 1979

Expected births	Registered births in the district	Per cent of district births registered
National crude birth rate = 50 per 1000 population		
District population = 156 000		
Expected births in the District = 7 800	2 109	27%

What are the health problems?

It is the serious diseases (as well as accidents which are common and either treatable or preventable) that are most likely to yield best results in response to intervention programmes. In children, nearly 40 per cent of the mortality is due to the major three diseases – malnutrition, respiratory infection and diarrhoea. About two-thirds of the mortality is due to the dominant nine which include the above three together with anaemia, tuberculosis, malaria and other parasitic diseases, whooping cough, measles and other common infectious illnesses of childhood, as well as accidents and poisoning.

In mothers, health problems surrounding childbirth are likely to be of major importance, particularly nutritional deficiency, anaemia, malaria, puerperal sepsis including tetanus and obstetric accidents. In adult males, communicable diseases, particularly tuberculosis, nutritional deficiencies and accidents may be important.

However, in no country's statistics is it ever mentioned that the main health problem is 'Lack of Services', especially in rural areas and for the urban poor.

The key questions for the District manager are 'How can one find out which of these problems are important in a particular District' and 'How can appropriate services be developed to deal with them?'

Finding out about health needs

Vital statistics and morbidity data have been used traditionally to assess health needs. Thus, rates of infant and pre-school mortality, perinatal and maternal mortality and rates of deaths from specific diseases (for example, tuberculosis) have been used as a measure of the health status of the population. Unfortunately, in most developing countries exact vital statistics at the District level are non-existent. Births and deaths may not be recorded, and many illnesses are never brought to the attention of the health personnel. In such cases one can make a start by making estimates from national data if available, or go by any information or indicators reported in the literature on defined communities in the country. Alternatively, it may be possible to carry out a small scale study in one or more randomly selected villages in the District in order to get some impression of probable rates.

In one community in Madang Province in Papua New Guinea, some nursing sisters at the Catholic Mission on Manam Island obtained as much information as they could on all the deaths on the island which came to their attention in $5\frac{1}{2}$ years (July 1971 to December 1977, omitting 1974). The total deaths recorded indicates marked under-reporting but even then their data represent a much higher proportion of the expected deaths than is normally found from records of health units. Table 2.5 shows the data they collected. Childbirth accounted for the death of 4 women out of the 151 adults recorded, 3 per cent of adult deaths. Unfortunately we do not know the number of births in this $5\frac{1}{2}$-year period so we cannot calculate the maternal mortality rate exactly, but the figures show that maternal deaths are a very important problem in this area as in many others. Deaths are also important because where there is one death there may be several other people severely ill. Problems following childbirth such as severe anaemia, vesico-vaginal fistulae, infection and perhaps infertility, are likely to be more common when there are deaths in labour. The opposite is also true.

The various sources of data available in the District need to be used carefully if we are to find out the true picture of illness in the community.

Table 2.5 **Causes of death on Manam Island, Madang Province 1971–1977** (omitting 1974)

Adults (N = 151)	%	*Children* (N = 88)	%
Resp. Dis. (incl. Tuberculosis)	34	Malaria	27
Old age	13	Resp. Dis. (incl. Tuberculosis)	23
Cancer	12	Diarrhoea	15
Accidents	7	Heart disease	3.5
Heart disease	5	Epilepsy	3.5
Childbirth	3	Accidents	2
Other	24	Other	26
Diarrhoea	2		

Source: Madang Province Health Team Report, 1979.

Certain problems will feature more in hospital statistics, others more in Health Centre data and some important problems we will only discover by visiting people at home.

In Madang District registered deaths among adults and children at the District Hospital are reported separately as in table 2.6. It was found that a very high proportion (44 per cent) of child deaths occurred in the perinatal period.

Table 2.6 Causes of death in Madang Hospital recorded on death certificates (January–December 1977)

Adults (N = 118)	%	*Children* (N = 108)	%
Pneumonia	21	Septicaemia	12
Chronic Lung Disease	11	Pneumonia	10
Tuberculosis	8	Meningitis	10
Trauma	8	Trauma	5
Heart Disease	7	Gastroenteritis	4
Renal Failure	5	Malaria	3
Cancer	5	Malnutrition	3
Liver Disease	4	Perinatal	44
Other	3	Other	9

Health centre deaths reveal the seriousness of chest infections

In Madang District Hospital mortality data were supplemented by information on deaths at Health Centres (see table 2.7). Pneumonia was clearly a far greater problem in the community than had been indicated from the hospital data. It now accounted for 44 per cent of child deaths at the Health Centre, compared with 10 per cent of child deaths at the hospital. There were also more deaths at the Health Centres from diarrhoea, and malnutrition was associated with 13 per cent of deaths in addition to the 2 per cent where it was recorded as the primary cause.

Health Centre attendance or discharge data reveal high prevalence of diarrhoea, skin problems and abdominal pain and a higher frequency of malaria, bronchitis and trauma

Data on deaths only give a partial picture of the diseases prevalent in the community as a whole. In the Ghanaian district it was only when attendance data were studied from the Health Centres that the widespread problems of diarrhoea, skin disease and abdominal pain became apparent besides malaria and upper respiratory tract infections identified in the hospital earlier (see tables 2.2 and 2.8).

In the Papua New Guinea Health Centre, discharge data also revealed the

Table 2.7   **Causes of in-patient death in health centres, Madang Province (January 1975 – February 1978)**

Adults N = 161	%	*Children* N = 139	%
Pneumonia	21	Pneumonia	44
Tuberculosis	16	Meningitis	9
Cancer	10	Gastroenteritis	8
Liver Disease	9	Meningitis/Cerebral	
Chronic Lung Disease	7	Malaria	8
Gastroenteritis	5	Malaria	7
Meningitis/Cerebral		Anaemia	5
Malaria	4	Trauma	4
Meningitis	3	Liver disease	4
Asthma	4	Tuberculosis	2
Childbirth	3	Malnutrition	2
Other	18	Other	7

Malnutrition was associated with another 18 deaths (13%)

Source: Death certificates returned to the provincial office.

Table 2.8   **Top nine reasons for attendance at an outpatient clinic at Juaso rural health centre, Ashanti-Akim District Profile, 1979**

		% Total attendances
1	Malaria	31
2	Upper respiratory tract infections	15
3	Diarrhoea	12
4	Skin disease	7
5	Abdominal pain	6
6	Eye problems	3
7	Measles	2
8	Worms	2
9	Wounds	0.5

high prevalence of diarrhoea in children and showed malaria to be far more frequent than death certificates suggested (see table 2.9). In adults, the discharge data show the importance of malaria, bronchitis and trauma (in addition to the pneumonia and tuberculosis shown in the mortality data in table 2.7).

The above discussion shows that every recorded death and every clinic attendance represents the 'tip of the iceberg'. For every known death or attendance at a clinic due to a particular cause there are likely to be several individuals ill for the same reason in the community. Thus known deaths and attendances can only give a glimpse of the picture of disease in the community.

**Table 2.9   Discharge diagnoses from health centres (April 1978)
Madang Province, Papua New Guinea**

Adults (N = 174)	%	*Children* (N = 183)	%
Pneumonia	25	*Malaria	25
*Malaria	20	Diarrhoea	21
Trauma	10	Pneumonia	14
Bronchitis	8.5	Malnutrition	12
Anaemia	8.5	Measles	9
Abscess	8.5	Trauma	4
Sores and ulcers	5	**Upper Resp. Tract Inf.	4
Diarrhoea	5	Eye infection	3
**Upper Resp. Tract Inf.	3	Sores and ulcers	3
Cancer	2.5	Anaemia	2
Other	4	Other	3
	100%		100%

* Includes fever, fever/headache
** Includes cough, cough/fever
This table does not include 86 confinements.

Clinic statistics from hospitals and Health Centres are notorious in under-reporting certain conditions, particularly chronic sickness, non-acute and non-epidemic diseases. Sickness rates are higher in the community than are ever reported at health units but clinic data give us a first view of the pattern of ill health.

Where are the health problems in the district?

Very often ill-health clusters in certain places or communities or families. All front-line health workers need to be trained to always watch for this clustering phenomenon. This is what one nurse noticed in the course of her work in a peripheral health unit in Malaysia (adapted from *The use of epidemiology by front-line workers in developing countries*, World Health Organization SHS/SPM/81.3. 1981).

She had noted from the weight-for-age charts that there were six young children with undernutrition in her area. These children all came from two villages which were situated on rubber estates in her area. The other two villages in her area had no undernourished children.

She investigated the families of the undernourished children and found that, in most cases, both father and mother were rubber tappers who left for work early in the mornings. Their young children were left in unsupervised nurseries where they were only fed milk from baby bottles if they cried. The milk was prepared by the mother before she left for work and was not properly refrigerated. The children frequently suffered from diarrhoea. From her observations she made efforts to visit the nurseries, train the attendants and improve their hygiene and methods of feeding the children.

This health worker had asked the right questions.

What is the event? A child persistently below the 80 per cent line of weight for age.

Who are affected? Children of mothers who work as rubber tappers.

Where are the events? Two villages in rubber estates; children attending unsupervised nurseries.

When did the events occur? Continuing at time of contact with the community nurse.

Are these events usual? Not usual in other parts of the area.

Why have these events occurred? Working mothers, bottle-fed children, inadequate nurseries, infection and diarrhoea.

What are the key factors? Lack of understanding of hygiene and nutrition by nursery attendants.

The clustering phenomenon is best revealed by charting events on a map of the area. Community nurses often have the knowledge required to chart health events on a map or on a chart, to see whether they are concentrated either in space or in time, or in a certain type of family. And if they are, she asks herself 'Why?' For a tentative answer to this question, she uses other bits of information which are available to her 'Could it be that communication difficulties, or low family income, or illiteracy, or the presence of a particular illegal injectionist are influencing the events?'

Many districts contain a variety of geographical areas and breakdown of data by these areas may reveal important differences due either to geographical or socio-economic factors. Table 2.10 shows outpatient diagnoses recorded in a specimen week in April 1978, in Papua New Guinea. They were obtained by calling in daily rolls to the Provincial Health Team Centre from all Health Centres, sub-centres and aid posts. Records were obtained from all Health Centres and sub-centres and 60 per cent of functioning aid posts. Because a Health Centre's outpatient department performs a similar function for its surrounding population as does an aid post, the results have been combined. The returns are classified by coastal, valley or mountain areas. Upper respiratory tract infection was rather more common in the mountain area, sores and ulcers were high in both mountain and valley areas. Malaria was nearly always found on the coast or in the valley, probably on account of conditions being more favourable for the mosquito to breed. Trauma seemed slightly less frequent in the valley populations.

In the Ashanti-Akim District of Ghana far more malnourished children were found in one area (Nyaboe) than in the other four areas studied (see table 2.11).

Table 2.10 Where are health problems in the district? Outpatient diagnoses (expressed as % of patients seen in each geographical region) Madang Province, Papua New Guinea 1978

	Coast (2657 patients)	*Ramu valley* (1054 patients)	*Mountain* (985 patients)
Upper Resp. Tract Inf.**	12.5 ⎫	15 ⎫	21 ⎫
Pneumonia	4 ⎬ 24	5.5 ⎬ 20.5	3.5 ⎬ 30.5
Influenza	7.5 ⎭	– ⎭	6 ⎭
Sores and ulcers	16.5	25	22
Malaria*	25	24.5	8
Scabies	4	9	7
Diarrhoea	5	6	7
Trauma	4	1.5	5.5
Eye infection	2	2	1.5
Abscess	2.5	1.5	2.5
Other	17	10	16

* Includes fever, fever/headache
** Includes cough, cough/fever

Table 2.11 Where are the malnourished children? Survey of 5 areas in Ashanti-Akim district, Ghana, 1977

Arm circumference	*Agogo* (N = 599)	*Bompata* (N = 237)	*Akutuase* (N = 101)	*Ananekrom* (N = 60)	*Nyaboe* (N = 157)
≥ 13.5 cm.	75%	74%	65%	73%	59%
12.5–13.5 cm.	21%	19%	25%	20%	28%
≤ 12.5 cm.	4%	7%	10%	7%	13%
Total percentage ≤ 12.5–13.5 cm	25%	26%	35%	27%	41%

Census data, routine statistics and survey data, if available, can be used increasingly to identify areas of a district where health problems are more likely to occur. From such sources one may be able to gather indicators of 'social malaise' which are highly associated with one another and with specific health problems. Useful data and indicators may include the folowing:

Differences in female/male mortality rates in specified age groups.
Proportion of females/males literate in rural areas.
Attendance rates at specified levels in schools.
Median years of education completed, male and female.
Percentage of women heads of household (widowed, divorced, separated, or husband away for long periods).
Average number of children in women-headed households.

When does ill-health occur?

Many diseases are seasonal. In countries with dry and rainy seasons, each season may bring a different disease pattern. Meningitis may be rampant in a savannah dry season as in the cerebro-spinal fever belt of Africa, and malaria when the rains arrive. Often long-awaited rain is associated first with relief because crops will begin to grow, but then with concern as malaria increases and the mosquitoes breed in the puddles. Diarrhoea increases, too, as the drainage system cannot cope with the heavy downpours. The situation is exacerbated by the fact that for many communities the first rains also herald the beginning of the busiest time of the year in the fields planting the new crop. There is little time left to care for children at home. It is also often a hungry season with the new crop only just being planted and stores from the previous crop fast running out. Where food stores from the previous harvest are low, prices of food in the market are usually at their highest point. Knowing when ill health occurs, the high risk times of the year can be recognised and some of the factors associated with ill health identified too. In the example described above, one most effective intervention may be to increase storage capacity of food after the previous harvest so the length of the hungry season is reduced and people are less vulnerable to infection.

In Bangladesh, studies in Matlab Thana have shown seasonal changes in the price of rice, the agricultural wage and household stocks of cereal. In the hungry season, as household stocks declined, wages decreased and rice prices increased (see figure 2.1).

Why does ill-health occur?

When several people are in contact with a pathogen only some people become ill. The same is true at the community level, certain families become ill, and in certain areas more people and families become ill than in others. By looking at these patterns in place and in time some of the factors associated with ill health begin to become apparent.

Interaction of nutrition and infection

It is well recognised that a large proportion of morbidity and mortality arises from the interaction of malnutrition and infection. The malnourished individual cannot muster an adequate immune response to fight infection. Hence even minor infections can spread, causing generalised disease in an organ or a system. Recovery is prolonged and may not be optimal. On the other hand, all infection has an eroding effect on the lean body mass causing loss of nutrients. The nutritional cost of repair tends to be heavy and the local diets are often incapable of meeting all the energy needs of the convalescing

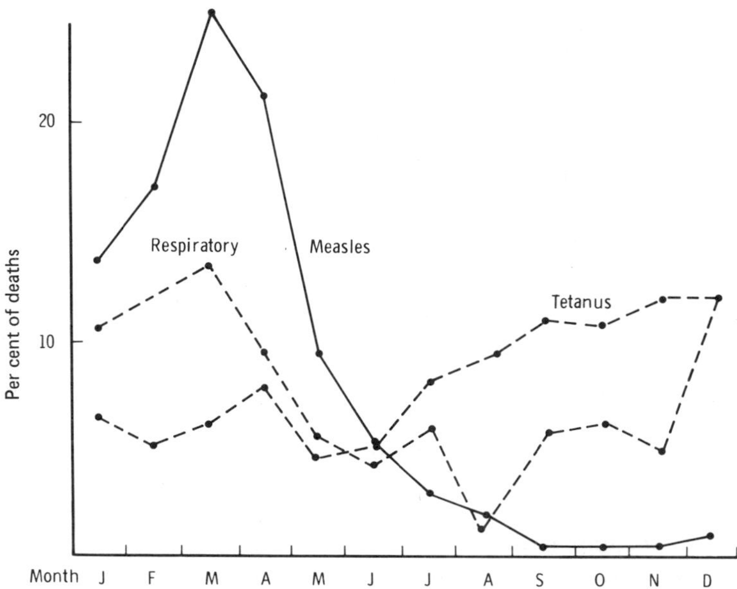

Per cent of child deaths (0-4 years) due to tetanus, measles, and respiratory
diseases by calender month

Figure 2.1   Seasonal mortality in Matlab Thana area, Bangladesh, 1976

Source: Sowie, Chen, L. C. Rahman, M. Sarder, A. M.
Int. of Epidem. (1980).

patient who may not have fully recovered his appetite. Moreover, the high
frequency of infective episodes results in a nutritional deficit from one illness
being carried over to the next. This accumulation of deficit after repeated
infections is best seen in children in the form of growth failure but also occurs
in adults. Hence control of infection and improvement of nutrition needs to be
a major objective of the district health programme.

A convenient approach to the control of some infections is through
immunisation. Both whooping cough and measles are serious illnesses of
children with high case fatality rates as well as causing serious and prolonged
weight loss. The treatment and rehabilitation costs of tuberculosis and
poliomyelitis are high and prevention through vaccination has been shown to
be cost-effective.

After measles and whooping cough, diarrhoeal disease is an important
aetiological factor in childhood malnutrition. Here early institution of oral
rehydration results in diarrhoea causing only a minimal disturbance in the
child's health. The illness is less acute and appetite is preserved. Early
institution of feeding helps recovery. Provision of facilities for oral rehydration at the village level has resulted in reduced morbidity and mortality as well

as an understanding of the fluid and nutritional needs of the patients.

A mistake in the past has been the failure to recognise the important role of infection in the aetiology of malnutrition. Nutritional status had come to be equated with nutritional intake alone and hence animal protein was awarded an important place. Energy intake and infection received only passing mentions. Now poor energy intake has been rightly recognised as being significant in the aetiology of malnutrition. And so also is infection. Hence the provision of adequate food and energy as well as control of infection must be integrated in all nutrition programmes.

Nutritional problems in developing countries

The major nutritional problems of protein-calorie deficiency, anaemia, blinding malnutrition, specific vitamin deficiencies and endemic goitre are now recognised. Of these, protein-calorie deficiency and anaemia are the most prevalent and have far-reaching effects on the health status of the community. When food is scarce, almost the entire family suffers from deprivation, but in general the effects are more devastating in those who are biologically most in need of food viz. the growing child, the pregnant and lactating women, and the convalescent. Some traditional diets have high roughage content and consequently low calorie density. This can cause problems with weaning foods. For example, some traditional weaning foods provide 1 kcal/g. of food compared to breast milk which has the energy density of 6 kcal/g. dry matter. The beginning of most childhood malnutrition can be traced to the weaning period. The slowing of growth in the first year of life accounts for 91 per cent of the deficit in body weight and 98 per cent of the deficit in length seen at the age of three. The low calorie density of some traditional food is also a limiting factor during convalescence when rapid catch-up and restoration of lean body mass is essential. But anorexia and weakness prevent the sick child from eating adequate amounts. A nourishing diet with adequate calorie density is also especially important at this period. One way of increasing the calorie density of foods is to add fats and edible oils in cooking. Red palm oil, coconut, cotton seed oil, ground nuts, soya and other sources of high energy foods are important nutritional resources which have been hitherto ignored because of preoccupation with animal protein.

Growing of food and its consumption is one of the most basic human activities. It is influenced by the laws of demand and supply as well as distribution, as is the case with every productive activity. Distribution of foods between and within countries, between rural and urban areas and within the family is sometimes as important as biological considerations of composition, methods of cooking, and so on. Rural health programmes need to take this aspect of distribution of an important resource into account. In most cases intervention is needed at the community level in addition to that at the level of the family and the individual.

Role of parasitic diseases

Malaria is ubiquitous in all countries of the tropics and the sub-tropics. In the early months of life the infant is relatively well protected because of the transplacentally-derived maternal antibodies. But as their effects wane, the infant and the young child become increasingly susceptible. This is therefore the age during which the main brunt of malaria is felt. In countries like Sri Lanka and Mauritius where effective malaria control programmes have been carried out, child mortality has been reduced by as much as half in some instances.

Another group in whom malaria is a serious problem are the pregnant women. Due to changes in the immune response caused by the hormonal changes in pregnancy, many women become increasingly vulnerable to malaria. Anaemia of haemolytic type is common and interferes with placental growth and function. Moreover, heavy placental infection by malaria parasites is also common so that low birth weight is a common complication of malaria. Infant mortality is closely related to the birth weight of the baby, the influence of which on survival can be identified up to the age of six months and beyond. Thus, malaria is an important factor in infant and child mortality.

In the adult, the main effects of malaria are in the form of chronic anaemia, lack of energy and vitality, together with a feeling of being unwell and increased susceptibility to infection because of compromised body reserves.

Other parasites

Similar reasoning applies to the effects of other parasitic diseases. Their effects depend upon the age and nutritional status of the host, the size of the parasitic load and environmental influences. Thus, even though a considerable number in a defined community carry a parasitic load, only a proportion suffer disease. From the disease point of view, the important parasites are *Entamoeba histolytica, Giardia lamblia, Ascaris lumbricoides, Ankylostome duodenale,* together with *Necator americanus, Strongyloides stercoralis,* and schistosomiasis. Infection is widespread, and so by comparison they constitute a large proportion of disease of parasitic origin seen. Many of the parasites have a complex life cycle utilising one or more intermediate hosts and their control will often involve control of such intermediate hosts as well as dealing with the reservoir in the community.

Determinants of disease and the physical, social and cultural environment of the individual

Mortality and morbidity figures convey only factual information. They cannot tell about the causation of disease and its determinants which often lie within the physical and socio-cultural environments and within the life-styles of the people. If health services are expected to help reduce the incidence of disease instead of being just palliative, then it is essential that the determinants of illness in the community are identified. Information obtained from morbidity and mortality statistics needs to be supplemented with other studies or surveys and particularly observation. In addition, KAP (knowledge, attitude, practice) studies, nutrition surveys, household surveys, and also agricultural profiles can be useful. Such studies tell us about what people do, when and why. It is only through creating a sufficient data bank and reliable system of health information relating to the community that health programmes and activities become relevant.

A great deal of disease in developing countries is environmentally determined. Even though the physical environment is obvious like vegetation and its insect breeding sites, housing, neighbourhood, sanitation, geography, seasonal climate and so on, the social and cultural environments are equally important but less obvious. Man is very much the product of the immediate society which he in turn influences by contributing to its social, economic, cultural and political life. Such interactions occur both at the individual level and at the family level, the latter being the unit of society. Most countries of the Third World are in a process of rapid transition so that a process of change is going through many of the socio-economic and political-cultural institutions of these countries. For many people life-style is changing, bringing new habits and new ways of thinking. Social and cultural currents run through all communities and societies. The concept of disease causation, the divining of illness, the selection of the provider of care, the customs and practices related to child-bearing and child-rearing are all integral parts of the provision of services. A good knowledge of local practices and socio-political trends is essential for providing the kind of service that people will perceive as stemming from national roots rather than a foreign concept.

Underlying many of the environmental determinants of health are the common elements of poverty and inequality. In all societies inequalities exist. There are inequalities of resources, privileges, opportunities, education and mobility. Naturally, inequality in one area engenders inequality in a related area, resulting in a class structure. It is said that in any social group with an existing inequality, any new resource or service will be shared out in accordance with the inequality. Those who are well-off will gain more than those who are badly off, unless special steps are instituted to avoid such an imbalance at the time of planning the service. Several corollaries arise from this aphorism. The most important, from the point of view of planning health care, is that when great wealth exists in a society, there is also great poverty, and often the former contributes to the latter. More often than not, the health professionals are also members of the upper social class and unknowingly part of the existing inequality. In almost all countries, therefore, the Law of Inverse Care applies so that those in greatest need of services get the least. Hence, in designing and implementing health programmes there is a great need to cater for the needs of those who are excluded from, and marginal to, the mainstream of development.

WHAT IS WRONG WITH THE EXISTING HEALTH SERVICES?

Health services do not always work perfectly but when a new plan is drawn up people may forget this. Planners may assume that with a new plan all the problems have been taken care of. In fact, if the existing problems have not been recognised and faced, they will merely be perpetuated into the new system.

Many developing countries are still in a state of transition from colonial rule to independent self-government. The seeds of the administrative and social services were sown during the colonial era and were essentially based on a Western model of planning. Even though many scientific and social developments occurred during the colonial era, the services tended to become 'institutionalised' and never 'popular'. In the case of health, for example, at the time of independence a framework of Regional and District Hospitals existed and the concept of the Health Centre was just about gaining ground. After independence an important influence on planning has been the professional one. Many of the leading professionals had received their specialist training abroad and were naturally deeply committed to the establishment and perpetuation of their own speciality. The result has been a continuing emphasis on 'curative' care based on hospitals and discrediting of the promotive approach in rural areas. This disparity between curative as against preventive/promotive medicine also permeates medical education which is largely based on curricula developed by medical schools in the West. In the case of the latter, public health and preventive medicine are often taught as postgraduate disciplines whereas in developing countries the need for teaching those subjects in the early years is obvious. Moreover, the practice of public health in a predominantly urban, literate, and technologically advanced society is so different compared to that in a predominantly peasant society though the principles may be the same. The district medical officer is a product of this system of health planning and education and will have to make continuing efforts to learn and match his skills to the problems in rural and peri-urban areas.

Are the services coping?

This question should be continually in the minds of all those who are responsible for providing services. The creation of health facilities and services does not in itself make a health programme. The activities of some of the services may be totally irrelevant to the health needs of the people.

Coverage (Are the services adequate?)

The main issue is that of coverage, and this gives rise to several subsidiary issues in the politics and sociology of health.

Several studies in different countries show that the large urban hospital serves the need of the educated élite but fails to meet the needs of the rural people as well as those of the 'fringe people' living in urban slums, shanty towns and inner city areas. The present curative system of health care has been correctly described as 'importing from abroad yesterday's solutions for tomorrow's problems'. A new approach and thinking are necessary for creating appropriate services to meet the needs of family health in developing countries.

With regard to providing coverage, *geographic coverage* of all areas of settlement in a district is important. In most countries provision exists for one rural Health Centre for every 100 000 population and a sub-centre for every 10 000. The geographic location of these health institutions is important since in practice most rural health units are accessible to people within a five-mile radius. They cannot be expected to provide effective coverage beyond this area. Whereas the sick can be expected to travel long distances for relief of pain or symptoms, services for the healthy must be delivered to them as near to their homes as possible. This is especially so with regard to services for women and children. The pregnant woman cannot be expected to make a round trip of more than six to eight miles on foot, often with a toddler in tow. Hence antenatal services and under-fives' clinics need to be organised at a greater number of places and not restricted to only Health Centres and sub-centres. Ideally these clinics should exist for every large village or cluster of hamlets.

Still on the subject of coverage, the frequency with which the antenatal and under-fives' clinics are organised will enable the people to make greater use of them. A clinic that operates on a weekly basis provides more effective coverage than the one operating on a monthly basis, and a daily clinic will be more effective than a weekly one. This ideal may not always be possible and a compromise formula may be needed in which clinics operate in rotation in such a way that on any given day a clinic is available within a four- to five-mile radius of every home in the District. Outreach or satellite clinics not only help to extend coverage, but enable the Health Team of a Centre to visit front-line health workers regularly and help to train them and upgrade their work.

Are Mother and Child Health (MCH) services being provided?

In most developing countries mothers and children constitute up to two-thirds of the population of an average District. They also constitute the biologically vulnerable groups. Hence Mother and Child Health (MCH) services constitute an important area of health care. Deficiencies or absence of any of the following basic health activities necessary for providing coverage in MCH

shows problems in existing services which need to be rectified before trying to
extend services further. For example, if midwives currently do not recognise
high risk mothers, how can they be expected to train Traditional Birth
Attendants (TBAs) to do so?

Basic activities in Mother and Child Health (MCH)

(1) Screening of expectant mothers. Identification of those at risk or with
abnormalities and their referral for more expert care.
(2) Assistance during delivery and puerperium.
(3) Screening, regular health surveillance and immunisation of children.
Identification of high risk families and further care of such families.
(4) Simple recording of health events in individual children, using a
weight chart. Data collection and evaluation.
(5) Health education emphasising nutrition, child-rearing, immunisation
and fertility problems.
(6) Providing information on community health problems to other
agencies and workers in the area and also to the community itself.
(7) Counselling and assistance with family planning.
(8) Distribution of simple medicines, food supplements and contra-
ceptives.
(9) The recognition and primary management of the most common
diseases in the area.
(10) Participation in the control of the communicable diseases through
immunisation, through diagnosis and treatment of index cases as in
tuberculosis, or through treatment of a reservoir of disease as in mass
de-worming.
(11) Liaison with community development, agricultural extension, education and other similar services in the area.

On these core MCH activities further services may be added, depending upon
local needs. For example, nutrition rehabilitation centres, mothercraft classes,
demonstration vegetable gardens, and so on. Adult literacy, especially female
literacy, has an important bearing on the health of the family and several
countries have integrated programmes of adult literacy with MCH services.
Based on recent experience in Sri Lanka and Kerala, it has been suggested that
for every one year of average schooling of girls, a reduction of 10 percentage
points in infant mortality can be reasonably expected.

Are people utilising the services?

Many people are reluctant to make use of medical services. This was thought
to be largely due to ignorance or cultural beliefs, but other factors play a part
too. For example, Health Centres and sub-centres stand out as different from

other constructions and dwellings in rural areas. Their style of construction, roofing, and the finish are different and most are fenced in. The health workers inside them are in uniforms and usually are people who were born in some other part of the country. They have a different life style and rarely do they participate in the social and cultural life of the village. Naturally the villagers are reluctant to 'intrude' on them. Attendances have been improved in many cases by 'localisation' of institutions through renting buildings rather than putting up new ones. Use of auxiliaries who are local residents and of village health workers as well as 'volunteers' from the local population also helps to remove local fears.

Community involvement at all stages – planning, implementation and evaluation – has an important effect on utilisation of health services. Involving the community demands continuing dialogue with the community and the establishment of village health committees. It is in these committees that most of the administrative and managerial problems can be aired. The health committee brings its own rewards usually through making local resources available, for example, a local building for holding clinics, selection of village health workers and their remuneration, volunteers and supervisors for health campaigns and sc on.

Health surveillance of vulnerable groups requires more administrative and managerial skills than specialised medical knowledge. Many non-medical individuals in the community who are literate and can communicate well are able to help in several ways. In the clinics they can assist with weighing and recording and in being the first contact with parents. The village teacher or social worker can help with home visiting and counselling. School children, by their involvement with school gardens and preparation of school meals, are a medium through which village schools can contribute to better eating habits. Indigenous midwives and even traditional practitioners have been enrolled to help in some cases. All these groups can generate a community interest and help improve attendances. Such use of available local resources represents an important element of the Primary Health Care concept. It enables community health programmes to be put into effect without undue delay.

Is the 'at-risk' concept being used in provision of health services?

The MCH team needs to select individuals and families 'at risk' of ill health for special care besides providing regular health surveillance of mothers and children. For example, the antenatal clinics are meant chiefly to provide the basis for healthy motherhood and not to diagnose obscure disease. According to criteria established by a simple study of local records, mothers may be selected for special care from among those attending the clinics. There will be a *primary selection* depending upon the obstetric and personal history of the mother, for example, very young, poor obstetric history, past history of complicated or instrumental delivery, history of stillbirths and neonatal deaths, failure of lactation with previous children, maternal height of under 5 ft (150 cm) and so on; and there will be a *secondary selection* depending upon disease processes occurring during the course of the pregnancy, for example, hypertension, toxaemia, anaemia, or social problems at home. In the same manner, the under-fives' clinic is meant for growth and nutrition supervision of the children and prevention of illnesses such as whooping cough, diphtheria, tetanus, poliomyelitis, measles and tuberculosis. From these clinics children may be selected for special care according to the following criteria:

(1) Broken homes, death of one parent or lack of parental care.
(2) Onset of another pregnancy in the mother.
(3) Failure of lactation.
(4) Multiple pregnancy, so that available breast milk is not enough.
(5) Low birth weight.
(6) Death of siblings.
(7) Presence of chronic illness in the family.

The special care provided may consist of more frequent visits to the clinic, home visiting, nutrition rehabilitation and health education, supply of food supplements, family planning or referral to other social services in the community.

Is there adequate quality of care?

The type and quality of care provided can influence the determinants of disease in the community. For example, when all Health Centres and sub-centres become just the extensions of the hospital out-patient departments they can have no impact on the health of the community. And this in fact has been the case with many health institutions. Small scale time/motion studies will indicate how the time of different health workers is utilised, and appropriate modifications can then be instituted. Such a study of the auxiliary nurse midwife in health centres in India showed that she spends most of her time in assisting for curative care and very little time on preventive/promotive care. A similar time/motion study of time taken by community clinic attendants to diagnose and write prescriptions gave an indication of the time taken up for treating common complaints (see table 2.12).

Related to the question of the quality of care is a subsidiary question – Are the health services relevant to the health problems of the community? What modifications and changes can be introduced to help the services deal with the major health problems more effectively? For example, worm infestation may be a major problem. The vermifuges dispensed at the sub-centre, however

Table 2.12 Consultation time for common conditions observed during a period of 4 days in 15 community clinics in Ghana.

| | No. of Cases | | | |
Time (minutes)	Cough	Diarrhoea	Fever	Total (%)
5	9	15	15	39 (19.5%)
5– 9	33	44	38	115 (57.5%)
10–14	18	13	11	42 (21.0%)
15+	3	1	–	4 (2.0%)
Average time per patient (minutes)	8.6	6.5	6.3	7.1

Source: Amonoo-Lartson, R. *et al. Soc. Sci. Med.* (1981) *15A*, 735–41.

effective for the individual case, may have no effect on the 'reservoir' in the community. Advising building and using latrines can affect the problem only gradually. On the other hand, a mass campaign for de-worming can produce immediate results and help to build confidence for the construction of latrines. Similarly, in the case of tuberculosis, case-finding by sputum examination and treatment may have a greater impact on the prevalence of the disease than mass miniature radiography.

Is staff morale high?

An important element in the quality of care is the general morale of the staff. Regular meetings with the staff, help with administrative and professional difficulties, involvement in decision-making, a regular supply of medicines and professional support helps to improve the quality of the care they provide. When health workers in remote rural areas feel abandoned, on account of infrequent visits, irregular supplies and no opportunity to improve their knowledge, morale sags and the quality of the work suffers (see also chapter 3, pp. 67–101).

Do staff interact?

If the health workers in the District are to become a proper Health Team then there is need for them to get to know each other and each other's difficulties. Regular meetings, refresher courses and seminars go a long way to building up a team spirit. Also, if the District Health Service is to become a viable system then, like any other system, it needs two-way traffic. There should be a flow of professional and administrative support from the centre to the periphery and regular analysis of health problems and effectiveness of programmes in the opposite direction. The greater the interchange and flow of information and ideas within the system, the more sensitive it becomes to the health needs of the community.

At present the Health Centres and sub-centres largely function as mere conveyor belts feeding 'interesting' clinical material to the specialists in the hospital. Such a system of health care can hardly ever expect to change the health situation. A new attitude in health care delivery is essential, such that the action shifts to the peripheral units and to the front-line health workers. In such an approach the role of the District Hospital and its medical officers is more in the nature of being supportive, managerial and administrative. Medical, professional and community resources can then be harnessed to deal with determinants of disease in innovative ways to bring about change.

Is there regular health services evaluation?

In all health work, regular and continuing evaluation is an important aspect of the activity. It enables the health team to decide upon priorities, to select areas where intensive effort is needed, to identify problems and to choose those approaches which appear most likely to be fruitful.

The community should be actively involved in the evaluation and be represented at all meetings where evaluation is being discussed. Similarly, various groups in the community can be of assistance in gathering data for evaluation.

Besides being essential for health planning, regular evaluation has a further advantage. It provides a basis for establishing a dialogue with the community through which the interest of the people can be maintained and their co-operation obtained for further development of health activities.

The evaluation component must be incorporated into a health programme right from the start, and must be designed to yield information for decision-making both at the operational and the planning levels. This calls for a data collection system which is simple and relevant to the successful operation of the programme. The purpose of evaluation is to improve staff performance and not as a punitive measure.

IDENTIFYING LOCAL RESOURCES

To identify health care resources in the District, the same five questions can be asked – who? what? where? when? why? In any given situation resources can be classified under the three major headings of: people, time and money, in that order of importance. In many health activities undue emphasis is placed upon money, so much so that its availability has become the only deciding factor for the commencing of any programme. Another less known aspect of resource is that in many cases the resource needs to be developed and strengthened. In the absence of such a careful 'tending' of resource it may often degenerate into a liability. For example, a healthy population full of vitality and with community cohesion is an important resource for development. But a sick population divided amongst itself and apathetic is a liability. The same principles apply to other forms of resource also. Money well spent on effective health programmes based on sound epidemiological data can provide immediate results. On the other hand, if it is tied up in impressive buildings then annual recurrent maintenance costs alone will be a crippling burden for years to come. The resource of time well utilised is an investment in the future. But if time has been wasted in getting projects off the ground, then not only can it never be recovered, but during that period the population (and the problem) may have grown larger.

Who is providing health care? Who do people go to for advice? Where? When? At what cost?

Who gives health care and advice?

Many different types of people provide advice and health care. If a child is ill, it is often a neighbour or grandparent who is the 'nearest source of help' and who will be the first to discuss with the mother what care is needed. After consulting near relatives or neighbours, the next type of person approached about sickness in a family is likely to depend on what the family thinks are the causes of ill health and which services they think may be able to help (see figure 2.2). In many societies the next source of advice and care is the drug seller or chemist or traditional healer. Spiritual healers may be sought to use their skills for specific problems. Other problems may be taken to the Health Centre (see figure 2.3).

There is growing evidence of the use of this wide diversity of sources of information. In one small-scale study in Newcastle upon Tyne, mothers in a low socio-economic neighbourhood were asked what action they took when their child was last ill. Nearly all the mothers had discussed the child with a grandparent (or sometimes a neighbour) to decide whether the child was ill enough to warrant going to the family doctor. In a larger UK study it was found that many people go to a chemist's shop to ask for help and purchase lotions and medicaments to try to solve their problems. Only certain problems are taken to the formal health services. The same pattern is found in other countries too. Figure 2.4 shows who people consulted in the Punjab for specific conditions. Skin rashes and spots of all types and also tetanus were likely to be taken to folk practitioners, pneumonia was likely to be taken to private practitioners or occasionally to the health centre.

TYPES OF PRACTITIONER	BACKGROUND AND TRAINING	PROPORTION % OF ALL PRACTITIONERS	DIARRHOEA	FEVER	RHEUMATISM	RESPIRATORY INFECTION	WORMS	JAUNDICE	FRACTURES	SNAKE BITE	HEADACHE
ALLOPATHS	High School 1–4 years apprenticeship	15%	⊡	⊡	⊡	⊡	⊡		☐		
HOMEOPATHS	Follows a school that uses minute quantities of medicine	3·3%	⊡	⊡	★	⊡	★				
KOBIRAJ	Ayurvedic training in herbs, minerals and diet	15·3%	★	★	⊡			★	⊡	★	★
TOTKA	Use Ayurvedic, Yunani and Shamanistic methods	60%	★	★	⊡			⊡	⊡	⊡	⊡
OTHERS	Yunani and Fakirs	6%	★	★	★						★

★ Over 10% of practitioners considered the disease their speciality

☐ Over 10% of clients would visit the practitioner for this disease

Figure 2.2   Specialisation amongst traditional practitioners: Bangladesh

Source: Glimpse 1980.

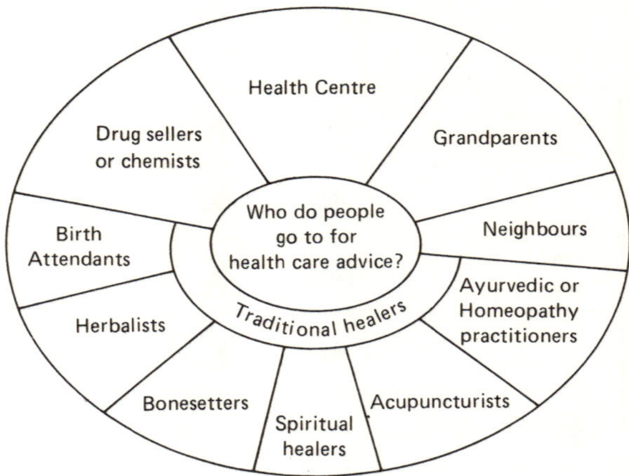

Figure 2.3   Who do people go to for health care advice?

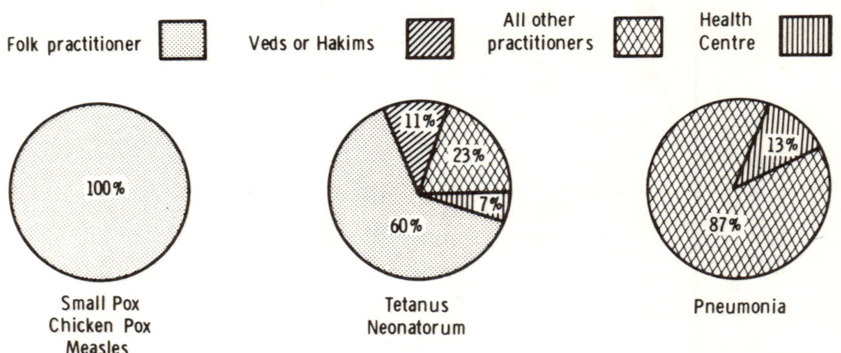

Figure 2.4   Who people consult about specific health problems (Punjab, India, 1972)

Source: Kaher *et al*. 1972.

In parts of Africa people prefer to consult a bonesetter for a compound fracture rather than go to the hospital. Where the causes of ill health are thought to be social and psychological, psychic healers may be consulted. Chronic illness is increasingly felt to be inadequately dealt with by the Western health system, and so when those suffering from chronic problems have tried the health care system, they may well try the many methods of alternative medicine. Many others feel the need to consult a health care provider who they feel understands their problems and background. Perhaps this is why hakims are in demand in West London and also why some Western women prefer to go to 'women's' hospitals or health care institutions.

Drugs are increasingly easy to obtain in many countries, from travelling drug sellers setting up stalls in markets and via chemists or drug stores. Many people are delighted to be able to buy what they need – family planning supplies, aspirin for headaches, and chloroquine for malaria. All these sources of health care are often far easier for most people to use than the health care system based in clinics and units often much further away.

Doctors, nurses, midwives, medical assistants, auxiliary nurses and environmental health personnel will all be providing health care in the district, some working for the government services, some for non-governmental organisations and others working privately. In addition to government health workers it is also useful to find out how many private health workers are in practice and also the number of non-government health units such as mission stations. These are resources with whom the district manager can often work in close collaboration.

In addition to *existing* staff some information is needed on future staff. One scheme for doing this is shown in figure 2.5. Such an analysis can lead to figures such as the following graph (figure 2.6) for Ghana. It shows a huge increase in enrolled nurses if projected to 1990 and only a very small increase in community nurses. When this was realised there was a policy change because it was community nurses who were needed for the future and not hospital enrolled nurses. Only by such analysis can underlying trends be recognised before difficulties arise.

Experience in several countries, chiefly in tropical Africa, but also in Papua New Guinea, Malaysia and Indonesia, has demonstrated the key role of the medical auxiliary for health work in rural areas. Yet the 1960s and 1970s were notable for the debate and the professional scepticism about the capabilities of such a person. The debate is now settled largely in favour of the auxiliary. A great boost to the concept came from the establishment of training programmes for the 'Medex' and the 'physician's assistant' in the United States. The debate in the present decade is about the part-time village health worker. This cadre is being trained and established as part of a national policy in many countries and in response to the call by the World Health Organization for Primary Health Care for all by the year 2000. For the doctor responsible for the health care of a District it will be more pragmatic to look upon the auxiliary, the village health worker, and the birth attendant as health resources, and to develop the quality of this resource through training and professional support as well as good administration instead of undermining their confidence through undue criticism.

National health plans are normally put together at the national level and the good ones make provision for manpower requirements on a national scale. District Health Teams will then have the responsibility of recruiting and

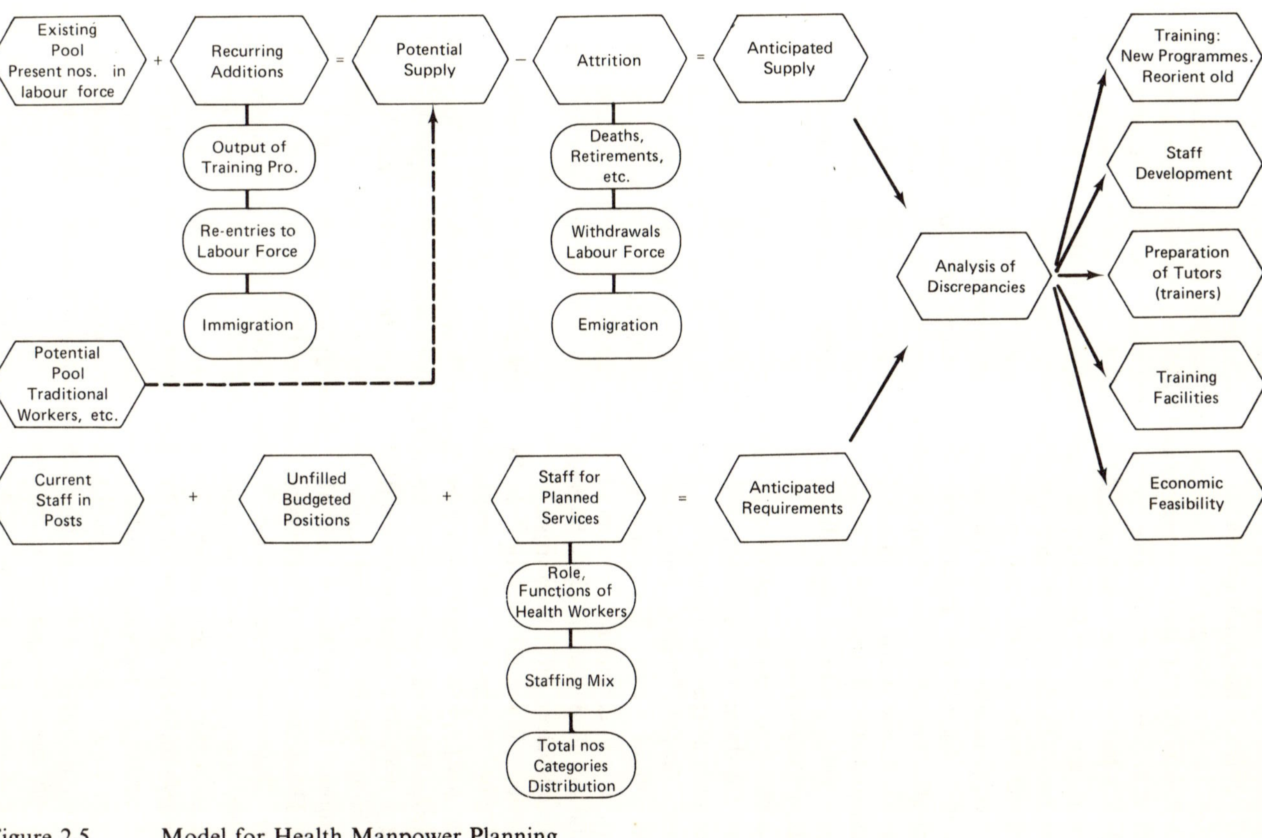

Figure 2.5   Model for Health Manpower Planning

Source: National Health Planning Unit, Project Team Spec./Human Resources, March 1978. Ghana.

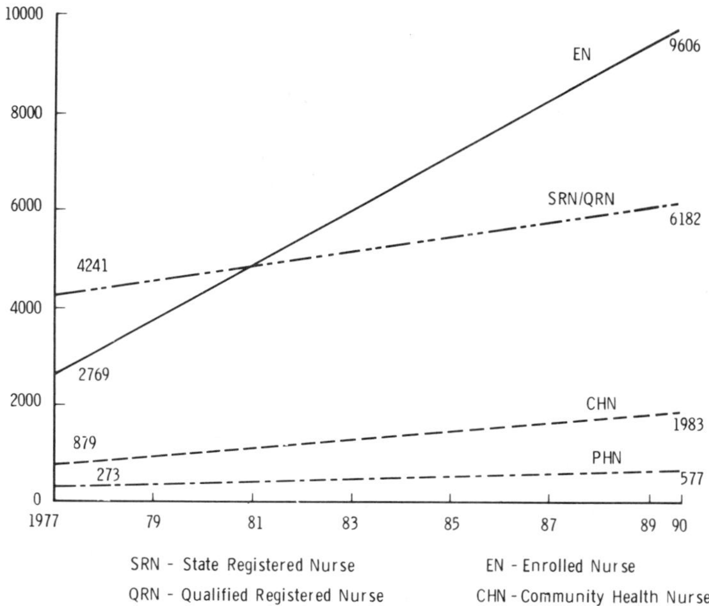

Figure 2.6   Projected supply of nursing personnel in active work in Ghana 1978–1990.
Source: National Health Planning Unit, 1978.

training front-line workers for carrying out health activities at the periphery. Professional and the higher auxiliary grades are usually recruited at the National level and trained at National or Regional health training institutions. At the District level, health manpower development must be more specific and task-orientated. In other words, the problems to be dealt with must be clearly defined, the tasks to be performed clearly spelt out and defined in detail and the staff required to perform them recruited and trained (see figure 2.7). The more peripheral the cadre of health worker, the more clearly defined should be the tasks to be performed to improve efficiency and effectiveness. Regular supervision and evaluation should be carried out to provide the background for a continuing programme of retraining and reorientation.

Where is health care provided and where do people come from to use it?

(a) *Where is health care being provided?*   Mapping Government and voluntary agency health facilities is most useful. Ordnance maps are available in most countries, and show the major towns and villages as well as roads, railways, rivers and other geographical boundaries. On such a map the District health facilities can be identified using symbols or coloured pins.

The district hospitals.   The District Hospital(s) plays a key role in a District's

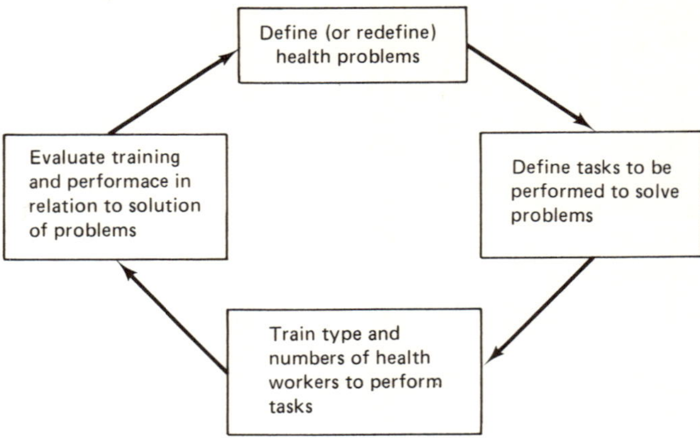

Figure 2.7   Assessing future staffing requirements

health care system if the latter is properly organised and well managed. Without the back-up facilities of the hospital, cases of complicated or advanced illness being referred as a result of increased health coverage cannot receive the special care they need, and the credibility of the health programme may suffer as a result. If traditional birth attendants are trained to screen for obstetric difficulties during the antenatal period, then facilities must be provided to deal with the referrals. This is good management. Emphasising preventive care does not necessarily mean that hospital care is to be neglected. In fact prompt treatment will often reduce the severity of illness. On the other hand, emphasis on preventive care is essential because it has not received importance in the past and because many illnesses are preventable. A good way of planning for the hospital needs of District health services is to compile a list of common medical, surgical and obstetric emergencies treated at the hospital. A review of admission registers and a few questions to hospital-based doctors and nurses will help generate such a list. Such an exercise will indicate the basic equipment and facilities needed at the District Hospital. In many places hospital outpatients and casualty departments provide the first point of contact for people seeking health care. Primary care provided only at the hospital is extremely expensive and an abuse of resource. It also leads to swamping of services so that the hospital workers are unable to look beyond the immediate problem of dealing with the crowds. They have no time left to see what is happening in the community.

(b) *Where do people come from to use health services?*   A rough idea of the areas served by a health unit can be obtained by recording the names of patients' villages as written in the out-patient register for every tenth attendant in a certain time, perhaps one year. This was done for the period 1 November 1968 until 31 October 1969 at Nkhata Bay District Hospital, Malawi. It was found that 47 per cent of out-patients came from within 1 mile (1.6 km) and 61 per cent from within 2 miles (3.2 km), 79 per cent came from within 5 miles (8 km) and 91 per cent within 10 miles (16 km). This decline in attendance with increasing distance is well known. In Tanzania it was found that up to 90 per cent of the patients come from within a radius of 5 miles.

However, this 'concentric circle' model of average attendance rates for all villages does not tell the whole story, since it is so dependent on population density. People obviously will travel further where routes are easier and transport readily available. One way of identifying the actual geographic range of a health unit is to calculate the percentage of the population seen for first attendance at an out-patient clinic; lines around areas with similar attendance have been called 'iso-care' lines (King, 1966). These are shown for the Nkhata Bay District Hospital in figure 2.8. The lines appear to follow the roads and the lakeshore very clearly. This confirms that communication (by road, or canoe on the lake) is very important for people when deciding whether or not to go to a health unit.

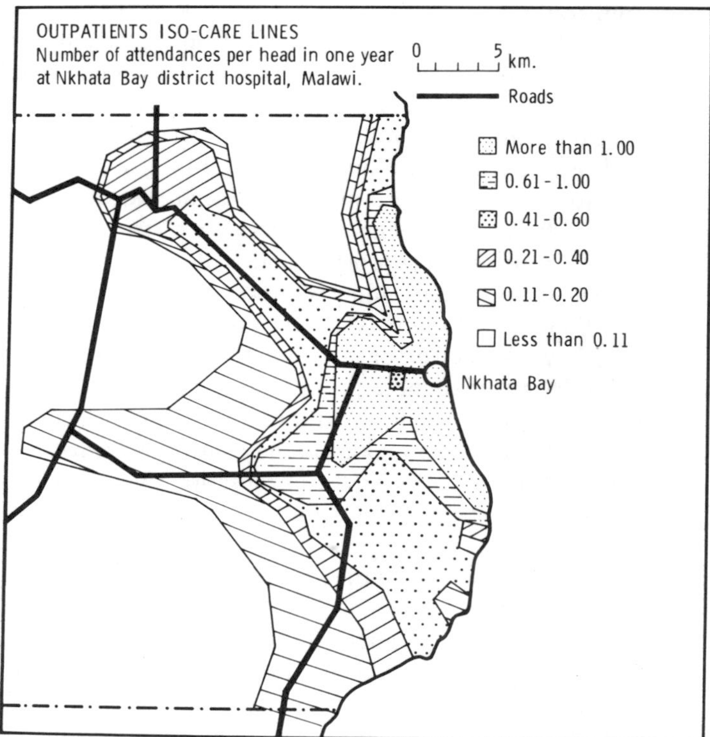

Figure 2.8   Catchment area, Nkhata Bay district hospital, Malawi

Sources: de Winter, E. R. (?1974) *Health services of a district hospital in Malawi*, page 110, Van Gorcum and Comp., N. V. Hubrecht Janssen Fund and Schiffner Fund, Amsterdam.

When is health care provided?

Are clinics held monthly, weekly, or do they never in fact happen at all? Is the time of day they are held just when most people go to the farm or to work? Are the times geared to market days and the availability of transport?

What health care is being provided?   (What range of services?)

One way of measuring what health care is being provided is to visit each health unit and find out when what services are provided. Another procedure is to go to traditional healers and their clients and ask them what conditions they treat or who they go to for specific help (see figure 2.2).

People other than health workers as resources

In every district a nucleus of professionals and para-professionals exists as part of the administrative and civil services. For example, in the health services there are District level specialists, general duty medical officers, nursing staff, medical auxiliaries and para-medical people. They have their counterparts in agriculture, water development, community development, road and communications, education and several other specialities. They form the technical-professional nucleus for activities within the district. Many of them also act as technical advisers to their counterparts in administration. Regular meetings of all the senior administrative and technical officers in a district are essential to integrate activities, formulate new projects and evaluate existing ones. For such meetings a right attitude to planning is important. In the words of Julius Nyerere, the function of the experts is to help people achieve the objectives they (the people) have decided upon and not to decide projects in closed meetings for them. However sound a project may be technically, the people will not make full use of it if they feel that it has been 'imposed' upon them. Involvement of people in decision-making at the political/administrative level is easier in countries with a policy of decentralisation. The idea is to shift decision-making to the District and Regional (Provincial) level instead of letting national and international experts in the capital city decide.

Away from the District administrative centre, technical help can still be found in the form of retired professionals and artisans. Many of them may be happy to do part-time work to augment their pensions. Thus builders, draughtsmen, plumbers, carpenters and many such artisans can be utilised for maintenance or extensions to buildings or for small-scale constructions. Protection and maintenance of wells and water tanks, or putting up new ones can be carried out with the help of such people who are not only cheaper, but also know the local conditions better than city-based specialists. In the Jamkhed project a local artist has been utilised to produce all the health education material used by village health workers. The drawings carry a good likeness to local features, clothes and habitats and are more effective compared to the bland material being put out by the national centre for health education.

Non-professional literate people can be identified in rural areas and encouraged to join as volunteer group leaders. Thus, plantations, mining concerns and small industries in many rural areas employ administrative and clerical staff. Shopkeepers and other self-employed people may be literate or possess skills which can be pooled together. Often their wives and other women folk may be literate or more enlightened than the general population. Such individuals can be encouraged to form volunteer groups for literacy, cooking, mothercraft or sewing classes or for organising child-minding and play groups. Such group leaders also need periodic training in becoming successful organisers and leaders and the District Health Team must take a special interest in organising such training.

Rural life is no doubt one of hardship but not necessarily one of failure against heavy odds. There are always some individuals who make a success of it. The successful farmer, the grain merchant, the successful cattle trader, as well as good parents, can be identified and persuaded to 'teach' others. Often these people have lively minds ready to adopt new ideas and equally ready to communicate new ideas to others. Communication of innovations is always a slow process in a traditional society. Where newspapers and others forms of mass media are relatively less important, oral communication remains the only way of spreading new ideas. In some villages of the Philippines, health workers have used village blackboards for spreading information and messages, but in the majority of rural communities oral communication is still the most important one. In this respect the village health worker is often an agent of social change because of the new ideas he/she introduces into the village.

Schools and school children can be developed into an important community resource. Each school child is a representative of a family and it is possible to teach parents and families through children. Furthermore, many school-age children participate in caring for their younger siblings at home and through them the care of the toddler can be improved. School children also participate in family activities on the farm or cattle grazing, protection of food crops from birds, harvesting and many others. Through them simple techniques like grain storage, soil conservation, composting, making soak-pits and so on can be introduced to families. Older school children can also become the nucleus of youth clubs, and instructions in good parenting can be organised for them. Finally, school buildings are important community institutions and can be utilised as focal points for community gatherings for seminars and study days. On such occasions the school vegetable garden can be used as a demonstration area.

The training institutions for medical auxiliaries and para-medicals are also usually to be found in the Districts. The students from these institutions can be utilised for small-scale community surveys which will be also valuable training for them.

People's skills are wasted if there is no channelling through careful community organisation. Formation of viable social institutions to support health programmes is often more important than putting up buildings for services. Here existing community groups can be approached. For example, in several countries of Africa the women's organisations are well developed and very influential. In countries with a one-party system of politics, the national political party has a great deal of social standing and is often active in social organisation. Local branches of such national organisations can be important allies in evolving programmes of health improvement.

Resources of material and labour

Many rural communities have traditions of mutual help. For example, in Indonesia such a tradition is well founded and often the village community gets together to help one of them with building, putting up an extension to a house, indoor work or other such activities. These traditions have been made use of by political leaders to promote national self-help schemes. Thus, the Harambe self-help schemes in Kenya have been responsible for setting up many local structures including large polytechnics. A very large proportion of Health Centres and sub-centres in Tanzania have been built through self-help schemes. More recently, in Jamkhed, India, self-help schemes have led to the construction of more than 20 small dams for water conservation schemes.

Besides resources of labour there may be other resources of material like wood (from local forests) and other products – stone (from local quarries), bricks (from local kilns) and so on which can be utilised for local activities, or as the focal point for setting up co-operatives and credit-unions. Such small scale economic institutions will provide further support for community organisation.

Amongst local resources special mention should be made of food resources. Since a large part of human productivity in rural areas is concerned with food production, it is as important to rural life as money is to a cash economy. With the present drive for cash crops the raising of food crops may suffer. Hence, conservation of the local food resource in the form of a proportion of land earmarked by every farmer for growing the family's food supply is necessary. Many countries have utilised the attraction of cash crops to create communal farms for growing these crops (while food is grown on the family plot) and to form co-operative unions.

With regard to growing food crops, the farmer needs to know what proportion of his land to allocate to the growing of staple food crops and how much to the growing of other foods to supplement these staple crops. In the past undue importance has been placed on protein foods, including animal protein. No doubt protein has an important role in the body's economy, but with increasing understanding of the role of energy in the diet, the raising of energy-rich foods will be an important step in the creation of local food sufficiency. Ground nuts and soya are important sources of energy as well as protein. Coconut, oil palm, sesame, mustard and other sources of edible oil like cotton-seed should be encouraged if the soil and climate are suitable. In this respect oversight can lead to a shortage of essential foods with a consequent drain of resources.

Whilst considering the preservation and further development of food resources it is important also to think of human milk as an important resource in child nutrition. Studies in many parts of the world have shown that even the average undernourished mother is capable of producing between 400–600 ml of milk in the second year of lactation. This would amount to an average of 300 mg IgA and 10 mg IgG per day in addition to the protein, energy and other nutrients. This important resource is being rapidly eroded under high pressure advertising of baby food manufacturers and needs to be conserved through control of promotion and by raising community awareness. Countries like Papua New Guinea, Burma, Algeria and Guinea-Bissau have passed legislation aimed at conservation of this important resource.

Financial resources

Financial resources in health are inadequate everywhere but particularly so in developing countries where the average per capita health expenditure is one US dollar annually. This low level of government expenditure on health is likely to continue in the foreseeable future. Therefore, for developing District health programmes, the main financial resource will have to come from rational redistribution within the health budget. Already disproportionately large amounts of money are being spent on large teaching hospitals so that in some countries the recurrent annual expenditure of the teaching hospital is equal to that of the total health budget of the country. In the regions, the expenditure on curative care, mainly through the Regional and District Hospitals is again unacceptably high, leaving very little resource for development of rural preventive services. It is the general rule with most services that once a pattern is established, any withdrawal of a service, however extravagant, leads to an outcry. Reallocation of funds for preventive/promotive programmes which can lead to curtailment of curative services is likely to be difficult unless backed by strong political decisions.

Under the circumstances described above, many health workers have looked for alternative ways of financing rural health services. These approaches have their advantages in that they make the village health services independent of the competing demands on the health budget. They also ensure a continuing high level of health awareness in the rural population to be prepared to contribute for their services. And people are more likely to accept without reservations and utilise those services which they have created themselves. On the other hand, methods of local financing do raise the moral issue that irrational use of curative services slanted in favour of urban élites will be allowed to continue and the rural poor must find their own resources for health care!

Many health workers have come up with innovative ideas for generating local financial resources. Credit unions and health insurance have been successful in Indonesia. The former consists mainly of a revolving fund concerned with productive activities like agriculture or cash crops. An agreed proportion of the fund is earmarked for health. In the case of the scheme of health insurance, households contribute a fixed amount annually towards health and in return receive free preventive services and subsidised curative care during illness. In the Sudan, when capital was needed for a new health activity it was raised by imposing a small tax on long distance bus tickets. More than enough capital was raised in a few years to help several other community programmes. In all countries where decentralisation has been the government policy, development programmes are decided at the periphery and funds are allocated accordingly. This does not necessarily mean that wise decisions will be made, because the disparity between curative and preventive care will continue unless fundamental policy changes occur. In many cases decentralisation only means a shift from projects in the neighbourhood of the capital city to projects in the neighbourhood of the Regional and District centres. However, it does also ensure that the District Medical Officer will have a say in the decision-making process. The success of his Community Health Programme, his ability to establish a dialogue with the people and to create a climate of thinking as well as his leadership qualities will help in the allocation of funds for relevant health activities.

Private sources like charitable institutions, local plantations or industries, including mines, and co-operative dairies may provide financial support for local health activities. Very often their contribution is limited to their employees and sometimes to the families of the employees.

Considerable savings in finance can often be made. In a one per cent sample of outpatient cards, prescribing patterns at one health centre in a district were analysed and the average cost was calculated. These actual costs were compared with a standardised regimen and large savings were possible (see table 2.13).

It was estimated that 'appropriate' prescribing could lead to a saving of 70 per cent of the drug bill.

Natural resources

The productive life and economic activity of any settlement or community is based on existing natural resources. Based on these resources, and the skills to

Table 2.13 'Actual' and 'appropriate' spending in primary health care

	Symptom as % of a 1% sample	Average prescription costs 'Actual'	'Appropriate'	Possible % saving
Malaria	51	0.57	0.23	60
Cough	17	1.35	0.12	92
Measles	4	1.38	0.68	51
Diarrhoea	3	0.79	0.54	32

Source: IDS Health Group (1978). *Health needs and health services in rural Ghana.* Institute of Development Studies, University of Sussex, UK.

exploit the resources, a whole pattern of life styles emerges with one activity dependent upon another. Thus, the presence of minerals may attract mining industry with its own technicians, managers and clerks upon whom in turn the local businessmen and farmers depend. These natural resources are therefore important for the survival of the community.

The most basic resources are land and water on which agriculture depends. Conservation of the community's resources with adequate and rational utilisation of land will help increase productivity. Similarly, water resources can be conserved and improved in a variety of ways. In most countries of Africa there is enough land in rural areas and land hunger does not occur as in several countries of Asia and Latin America. In Asia, up to 40 per cent of a rural population may consist of landless labourers dependent for their livelihood on the vagaries of nature and the whims of the landlord. This situation is even more desparate in some countries of Latin America where less than 1 per cent of landowners occupy 42 per cent of the cultivable land. Most of these large tracts of land are used as ranches and plantations and the smallholders, who are the real producers of food, may have very little land available.

Equity in land ownership and land reforms may be beyond the scope of the District Medical Officer. But establishment of small plots of communal land for demonstration and teaching agricultural skills, and the use of the produce for pre-school feeding and for local nurseries, is an important part of nutrition rehabilitation. Several programmes of community health have found it necessary to branch out into the training of village agriculture workers including simple veterinary skills. These activities not only help to generate a new resource in the form of training for the peasant farmer, but also sufficient produce to support communal feeding programmes. Community awareness of local resources also leads to care of the environment chiefly in the planting of trees and the prevention of deforestation. The quality of the community's life is closely linked to the quality of the environmental and natural resources. Their preservation can often be made part of the community's responsibility.

Methods for finding out what is happening in the district

There are five main ways of finding out about communities within a Health District:

(1) The first method is to make a checklist of information required for reasonable planning and delivery of health services bearing in mind the human, material and financial resources that will be needed. The information can be extracted from available health statistics and from knowledgeable persons both within and outside the community.

(2) The second method is the use of existing data and records of health and health-related institutions in the district.

(3) Another method is the use of household surveys to obtain the socio-economic characteristics of the community such as housing, income, major economic activities and sources of food and nutrition which may have a bearing on health. During household surveys, knowledge, attitudes and practices relating to health problems should be obtained to provide the basis for health education plans, programmes and activities.

(4) Very occasionally, clinical surveys may be useful to obtain information on the health status of the community. Although such clinical surveys are expensive, they may offer the only alternative method of knowing about the prevalence and specific symptoms of important disease conditions in the community. Essentially, clinical surveys represent mass-screening procedures and as in mass-screening procedures, steps must be taken to make some treatment available for common illnesses which may be brought to light.

(5) Mass physical examination for assessing the health status of a community has been used in community health research projects. Useful as mass physical examinations in small communities may be, they can be very expensive. On the whole, mass screening procedures tend to raise the expectations of people examined and one must be ready to treat cases detected immediately if people are not to lose interest in continued participation in such community health action programmes.

The community round

A simple but effective way of finding out, at a glance, the likely health needs of a community is to do what is appropriately referred to as a community round. A community round can provide the same assistance to a community health worker as the clinician gets when he goes round the ward to assess the health needs of his patients and to prescribe treatment. Dialogue and interviews with key rural persons is useful in identifying local needs. The natural and elected leaders in the community are often used as key informants and it is advisable whenever possible to work through them. However, it has been often said that many of them represent one point of view and may speak with vested interests.

In every society there also exist people who refuse to make use of the services, who disagree with the generally held opinions and are considered 'different'. Obtaining their views may also be of interest. Another group of key informants are the teachers. Teachers are keen observers of social and political currents in the community. Through their pupils they are in close contact with families and can often provide a balanced view of the community's needs as well as opinions about services. In every social group there are also individuals who are innovators and spread new ideas. It is important to identify such individuals and establish a regular dialogue with them. Also, as a method of obtaining reliable information 'group interviews' can be very helpful. When a person speaks in the presence of other community members, the information is likely to be more relevant and truthful on account of social pressure. The antenatal and under-fives' clinics provide many opportunities for such group interviews. Farmers' clubs, youth services and clubs, women's organisations and various religious groups are further examples of available sources for group interviews.

Why surveys may be required

There are three particular reasons why all illness is not necessarily reported to the health services. Many illnesses thought to be caused by evil spirits, breaking of taboos, or witchcraft will obviously be attended by the indigenous practitioners. Thus, in Uganda, kwashiorkor (obowesi) is thought to be due to jealousy between the child in the womb and that on the breast. Western medicine obviously has no cure for it and many cases of kwashiorkor are not brought to the notice of the medical services. In India, measles and several childhood exanthems are considered to be caused by the visitations of a deity and are not brought to the notice of the medical profession.

The second important reservation about health service morbidity data relates to the inverse care law mentioned earlier. Those in a community who need services most, utilise them the least. This is because they live too far away, or they cannot afford the fees, or they belong to a low social class, or they feel excluded, or have a major family discord causing unhappiness and depression, or the drudgery of earning a living leaves them with very little free time and energy to do anything else. Hence a special effort needs to be made to identify such groups and their most prevalent health problems in order to obtain a more complete picture of the pattern of ill health in the district.

Thirdly, in many countries where most diseases are acute, the morbidity data of health institutions mainly reveal attendances for such illnesses as was shown in table 2.8 and figure 2.8. It seems that chronic illness is not considered important enough by the people and the health profession alike to merit a great deal of time and attention. People may have learnt that little is done if they bring such problems to the health units. Thus, cases of established polio paralysis, cerebral palsy, blindness, and other handicapping or chronic illnesses are rarely brought to the health centres or hospitals for treatment. Visits to villages and surveys of pre-school and school children are essential to obtain information about the prevalence of such health problems.

The above reservations should be borne in mind when planning surveys. A key factor in their success is generating good questions, which requires the identification of key issues in a topic. An example of key issues in child feeding is given below.

Finding out about child (0–5 years) feeding

How do people feed their young children?
    Breastfeeding? Food and meals at different ages?
    Quantity offered and eaten? Energy density?
    Nutrient values? Frequency of feeding?

Are child-feeding practices 'satisfactory'?
    Identify the areas where problems are known to occur.

Why do people feed young children in the way they do?
    What do we see if we spend three days in each season
    observing and participating in local family life?

How much trouble would it be for people to change? What would be the cost?

What do people see as their main problems in feeding young children?

If people do change their behaviour, what will the consequence be? Will it work in their situation?
    What happens when mothers use a new weaning food and find their children have diarrhoea?

What do people think they will get out of changing?
    Prestige? Convenience?
    Healthy and attractive children?
    More productive children?

How are people changing their child-feeding practices already?
    What happens when grandmothers and daughters talk about the way each has fed (or is feeding) their children?

Another example of the use of surveys to assess prevalence is in the case of residual paralysis after polio. A postal enquiry to school teachers in areas where at least 70 per cent of children attend school has been shown to be an efficient method of measuring the prevalence of polio. This method first developed in Ghana has now been tested in several countries.

Surveys of health service delivery problems – operational research

In the actual process of delivering health care, it is important that procedures be constantly monitored to provide information for the reappraisal of desired goals so as to prevent programmes from being shipwrecked.

Operational research aims at applying management techniques for the improvement of health care delivery. In a way it is a method of on-site evaluation for staff engaged in the actual process of delivering health care without waiting for outside agents to detect faults after irreparable damage has been done.

One effective way of conducting operational research in clinics, Health Centres, health posts and other District and sub-district health institutions is the use of trained observers to administer appropriately designed questionnaires or check lists while observing processes resulting from the interaction between health providers and patients as well as other persons attending special sessions at health facilities.

When direct observation procedures as described above have been refined and standardised, it should be possible for health facility staff to conduct a retrospective audit of clinic records and institute immediate action to improve the running of their health facility.

In summary, the pattern of epidemic, acute and life-threatening disease can be obtained from hospital and clinic statistics. Information on the age distribution of the population can be obtained from local enquiry and confirmed from census data. When information is needed about the pattern of other prevalent illnesses, particularly chronic and handicapping conditions in rural areas where there are no clinics to provide even approximate statistics, a supplementary method for obtaining information is required. If the sampling technique of the survey is well designed, a small number of subjects will provide information representative of the whole group or area. Information on morbidity thus gathered can be further added to and improved by means of interviews with community leaders, other residents and practitioners. Surveys of practices and attitudes may throw further light on beliefs about disease. Naturally, this source of information is not available immediately. As gradually trusts and relationships get established, and friendships are built, more reliable information of this type can be gathered.

Resources can be identified by mapping existing health care facilities and staff. Enquiry will add the whereabouts of other practitioners in the district. Attendance can be examined to find out where people come from. Gradually information can be assembled on other resources affecting health and health care; people (in agriculture, education, and so on); equipment and time spent; natural resources, and so on.

FURTHER READING

Brown, J. E. and Brown, R. C. *Finding the causes of child malnutrition: a handbook for developing countries*, Task Force on World Hunger, 341 Ponce de Leon Avenue, Atlanta, Ga. 30308, USA. 1979.

Department of International Health, The John Hopkins University School of Hygiene and Public Health, *The Functional Analysis of Health Needs and Services*. Asia Publishing House, Bombay and New Delhi. 1976.

IDS Health Group. 'Health Needs and Health Services in Rural Ghana'. *Soc. Sci. Med.* (1981) *15A*, 397–495.

King, M. *Medical Care in Developing Countries*. Oxford University Press, Nairobi. 1966.

Potts, M. 'More marketing than medicine', *People* (1981) *2*, 6–7.

Werner, D. and Bower, B. *Helping health workers learn*, Hesperian Foundation, P.O. Box 1692, Palo Alto, CA 94302, USA. 1982.

World Health Organization. *Uses of epidemiology by front-line workers*, Offset series, WHO, Geneva. 1981.

3 Making a Health Plan for the District

There are clear advantages in developing a planning process. When there is a plan, action is required by specified people and lack of action is soon apparent. With clear aims and objectives people can be selectively involved to do specific tasks that need to be done. A good plan can consider many relevant factors and at the same time give a composite over-all view to numerous parts. Together with its unifying direction and purpose it can also encourage the use of a range of alternative strategies to find out which works best where. It can also be a medium for questioning and challenging traditional assumptions not only about what are the top priorities, but also about who should do things and how they should be done. With a plan, action is clearly defined with regard to specified problems and utilising specified resources, and can therefore be measured for its effectiveness in alleviating problems and its efficiency in terms of cost. Feedback can be obtained on how well specific aims can be put into practice.

WHAT IS A PLAN?

A plan is a course of action one intends to follow in order to solve a problem. It ensures that objectives are set to deal with problems and to make best use of available resources. A plan also provides the opportunity to consider all the options available for the performance of tasks in response to needs.

Planning may be thought of as a process both at the central and at the peripheral level. At the central or policy-formulation level, a plan considers the broad outline of what needs to be done and the resources that must be committed at the National level to enable policy objectives to be achieved. On the other hand, at the peripheral level, details of actual tasks to be carried out, and who is to perform them, must be considered in the face of real everyday problems of resources and organisational difficulties. Planning at the periphery, namely at the District or community level, needs to be more pragmatic and less conceptual than at the National or the Regional level.

Planning at the central and peripheral levels must not be considered as separate exercises because information obtained from the periphery is required for central planning. Similarly, national guidance and policy are also needed in peripheral planning. Planning based on needs identified at the periphery is sometimes referred to as the 'Bottom-Up' approach in planning.

THE PLANNING PROCESS

The health planning and implementation cycle

The essence of effective planning lies in finding answers to four key questions:

   (1) Where are we now? (District assessment)
   (2) Where do we want to go? (priorities, goals, targets, decisions)
   (3) How will we get there? (organisation and management)
   (4) How will we know when we arrive? (evaluation)

The steps in conducting a district assessment of health problems, resources and opportunities were discussed in chapter 2. Only when a searching assessment has been done can the next steps be taken. These are to establish health priorities; then to identify key tasks for action, their organisation procedures and required inputs, and to put the plan into action with built-in feedback mechanisms (see figure 3.1).

Dangers of planning and why planning sometimes fails

A formal planning system can have dangers as well as advantages, and these need to be recognised and avoided. One possible problem of 'over-planning' may be that there is little scope for flexibility and innovation after the plan is written. Alternative approaches for solving a problem may be forgotten in the bustle of making a decision to do something. Good ideas may have no mechanism for being brought forward and put into action. People may feel there is little scope for innovation and creativity locally. Another problem is that too many people may be involved. Alternatively, inappropriate people may be involved. This is particularly likely when planning is over-centralised and done without the participation of local people or the staff at the periphery who will be responsible for putting the plan into action. Another problem can be that an elegant plan can be completely misconceived and wrongly focused. The planning process can also absorb too much time so that most of the time

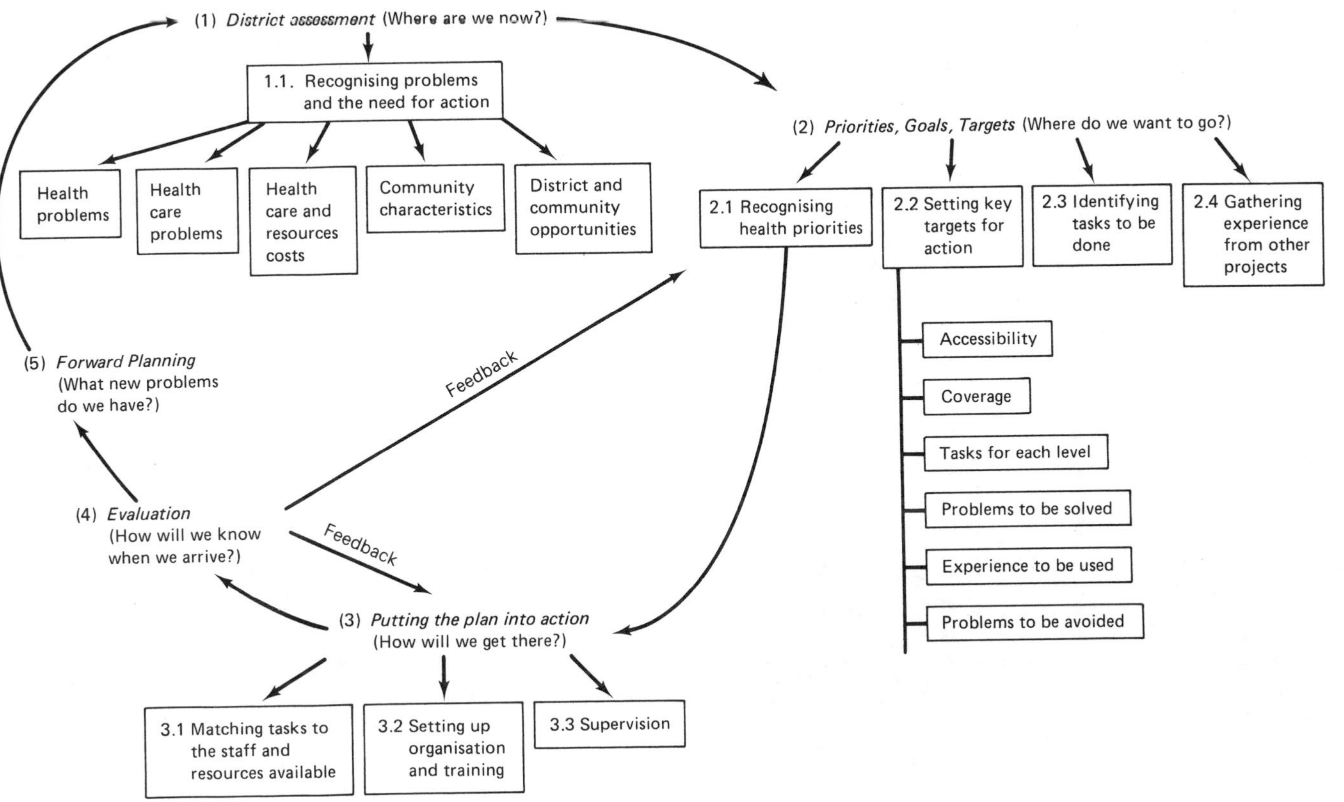

Figure 3.1   The health planning and implementation cycle

available is taken with drawing up the plan and there is no time left to tackle the important issues associated with putting the plan into action. When this happens it is easy to get strategies in the wrong sequence and if there is no flexibility in the plan this will cause considerable difficulties. Even though a number of problems can be envisaged with a forward planning system there are still many advantages in developing a planning process. These are compared with the pitfalls in table 3.1.

Table 3.1   Some advantages and pitfalls of formal planning systems

Possible advantages	*Possible disadvantages*
1 Action is called for; no action is immediately apparent.	1 'Over-planning' and inhibition of creativity and innovation, especially when front-line health workers and the community are excluded from the planning process.
2 More people selectively involved to do specific tasks.	
3 Many relevant factors considered	
4 Common or traditional assumptions challenged and questioned.	2 Too many people or inappropriate people involved.
5 Unity of direction and purpose.	3 Wrong focus.
6 Encourages use of a range of possible strategies.	4 Takes up too much time.
	5 Insufficient time available to plan properly.
7 Plan can be evaluated.	6 Curtailment of flexibility.
	7 Strategies may be considered in the wrong sequence.
	8 Plan may be too broadly defined to be measurable.
	9 Inhibits action on immediate problems.

(Adapted from Camillus, J. C. (1975). *Evaluating the benefits of formal planning systems, long range planning.*)

Plans may sometimes fail. It is by understanding why such failure occurs that planning processes and plans themselves can be improved. Table 3.2 lists some of the reasons why planning may fail. The three main reasons for failure are: (i) lack of commitment by key managers, (ii) poor planning processes, and (iii) plans remain on paper and are not implemented.

Planning is a learning process

Planning is a continuous learning process. Aims need to be constantly reviewed as the pattern of health problems changes, as opportunities arise for more effective use of resources, and as the focus of priorities and policy moves. This continuous process is illustrated in figure 3.2.

Table 3.2 **Why planning sometimes fails and what can be done**

Why does planning fail?	*What can be done?*
1 *Lack of commitment by key managers*	
1.1. Lack of acceptance by 'operational' personnel who will put the plan into action.	Involve 'operations' people in drawing up plans.
1.2. Lack of interest and commitment by senior personnel.	Ensure commitment before starting to plan.
1.3. Some managers are allowed to opt out.	Ensure involvement of all managers at an early stage.
1.4. Confusion about what 'corporate' planning means.	Get commitment to the District health activities by all segments involved in health and get all these views represented in the plans made.
1.5. Planners ignore the work people are already doing.	Find out what people do and the problems they have before recommending any change.
2 *Poor planning processes*	
2.1. Plans are made centrally in 'ivory towers'.	Hold discussions with people working at the periphery.
2.2. Confusion between strategic and operational planning.	Distinguish broad policy making and strategy from the details of putting a policy into action.
2.3. Trying to plan through committees.	Set up a working group instead.
2.4. The planner is of too low a calibre.	For negotiation find someone who is acceptable to most of the segments that will be involved in putting the plan into action. For the hard routine of working out the plan's implications find someone who will do the job well – they need not be the negotiator.
2.5. The planning system and the plan is too sophisticated and too complex.	Make it simple so it fits in with people's current work.
2.6. Planners fail to accept the limitations of their role.	Distinguish between planning and the 'operational' activities of putting plans into action.
2.7. Insufficient attention is given to the format of plans.	Use a simple format and seek the views of others.
3 *Plans are not used*	Implementation needs to be built into the plan. Commitment is needed before plans are drawn up, and maintained during implementation.

(Adapted from Hussey, D. (1974). *Corporate planning: theory and practice.* Pergamon Press.)

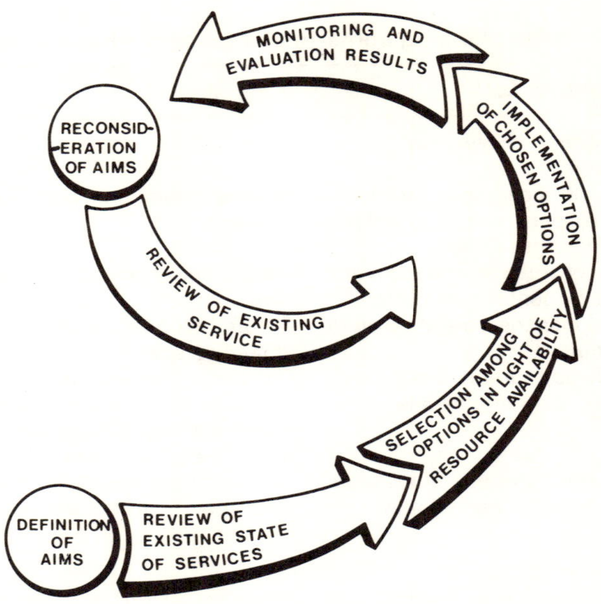

Figure 3.2   Planning is a learning process

Key concepts in effective district health planning

(i) *Priority health problems determine health service functions*

Once the priority health problems are recognised, and the conditions, causes and risk factors contributing to them identified, it is possible to define clearly what the functions of the health services need to be. As described in chapter 2, the priority health problems are selected on the basis of their prevalence, seriousness, preventability and treatability. Table 3.3 shows an example of priorities in planning for child health services. Naturally, when the health problems change, a new plan with new health service functions is needed.

(ii) *Health service functions determine what accessibility
to services is needed*

If health services are to provide care effectively, certain services (such as monitoring children's growth) need to be available very close to every home in the local community. Other services (such as blood pressure measurement during pregnancy) need to be within 4–5 miles (8 km) or two hours travel, possibly at a small health station; and for certain emergencies as well as for some specialised types of care, a District Hospital needs to be accessible, ideally not more than three hours travelling time away (see figure 3.3 and table 3.4).

Table 3.3 **Priority health problems and functions of health system: child health**

Priority health problems		Functions of child health services
	Basis for Selection	
Group 1: Malnutrition		Supervise and maintain health of young children by:
Malaria Severe chest in- fections, mainly pneumonia	different mixtures of prevalence, seriousness, preventability and treatability	(1) *Promotion of nutrition* – nutrition education on food needs and feeding practices (primary prevention of malnutrition) – supervision of growth and early detection of malnutrition (secondary prevention) – supplementary feeding when necessary
Measles	prevalent, serious, pre- ventable and/or treatable	(2) *Primary prevention of infectious diseases through*: – immunisation – prophylactic drugs (e.g. antimalarials, treatment of contacts)
Acute diarrhoea		– health education
Group 2: Neonatal tetanus Polio Tuberculosis	serious fairly prevalent but easily prevented	(3) *Management of common childhood infections (as above list) by*: – early diagnosis and effective therapy (including health education on early symptoms and home treatment)
Group 3: Intestinal para- sites Skin infections – wounds Conjunctivitis	prevalent, debili- tating preventable and/or treatable	

Source: IDS Health Group (1978). *Health needs and health services in rural Ghana*. Institute of Development Studies, Brighton, UK.

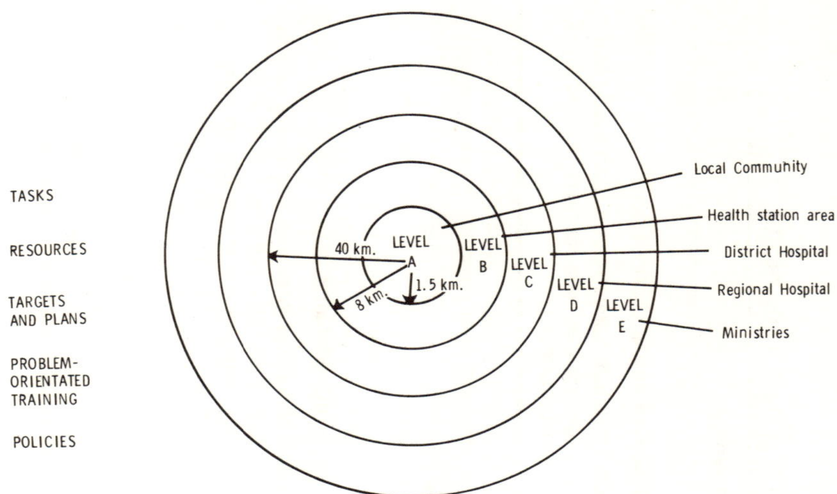

Figure 3.3   The over-all health care system with health functions determining
                    accessibility to services

(iii) *Health service functions also determine task definition and evaluation*

Once health service functions based on priority problems are recognised and
the accessibility of various services determined for each of these functions,
tasks can be defined as components of such functions. These tasks can then be
allocated where services are needed and with the resources available. Table 3.4
gives an example of task specification for the control of malaria. It also shows
the division of these tasks into three levels, the Local Community, the Health
Station, and the District. This task definition and allocation with the resources
available is in itself a tool for evaluation of what is being done. Moreover, such
an allocation of tasks takes into account the fact that the control of malaria
requires a number of health activities by different departments, including, for
example, environmental sanitation, health education, curative services, and so
on.

(iv) *Health problems require action on causes of ill health, early intervention and rehabilitation as well as cure*

Most health problems require action at several stages:

(1) *Health promotion* – to maintain healthy life-style.
(2) *Action on causes* of ill health before a health problem begins (for
    example, improvement of a household's eating patterns, clearing
    mosquito breeding sites, removing health hazards, providing
    immunisation).

Table 3.4 Control of malaria in a district

LEVEL A The Local Community	(1) Clearing breeding sites Burying tins etc. Draining swampy areas and waste water. Keeping eaves, water butts etc. covered (2) Distribution of antimalarials (and keeping records in family register) to under fives to pregnant women (3) Treatment of acute attacks of malaria and recording each episode in family register. Sponging for high fever Chloroquine tablets
LEVEL B The Health Centre	(1) Treatment of severe attacks of malaria referred from A (2) Drug supplies for Level A (3) Collect records from Level A (4) Spraying campaigns in local communities (5) Training for Level A
LEVEL C The District	(1) Treatment of severe cases referred from B (2) Monitoring incidence in district (3) Maintaining spray supplies (4) Maintaining drug supplies and teaching to 'B' and 'A'

(3) *Early intervention to prevent the problem becoming serious* (for example, health surveillance of children and pregnant women and early treatment of infections, recognising high risk mothers and children and families and providing special care).

(4) *Cure* if possible when the problem does arise (for example, proper care of the sick and injured).

(5) *Care and rehabilitation* after the problem has gone (for example, provision of aids for mobility for post-polio patients).

Figure 3.4 shows how the different types of interventions described above are intended to alter the prevalence and seriousness of a disease, in this case, anaemia.

(v) *Functions and task definition determine the pattern of staffing*

The aim in manpower planning is to get the right person in the right place at the right time at the right cost. By using task definition, a right person can be specified who will be able to do the needed job. When tasks have been specified, evaluation of what has been or has not been done is also made very

Health promotion	Health care	Prevention of anaemia	Early diagnosis and treatment	Spontaneous cure
				Death
Natural history of anaemia in the community				Chronic disability
Health education Individual and community measures for prevention of malaria, hookworm, etc. Adequate diets	Distribution of antimalarials to vulnerable groups De-worming Issue of dietary supplements, e.g., ferrous sulphate Screening for anaemia	Facilities for early diagnosis and simple therapy in the clinics Referral to hospital	Treatment and rehabilitation	

Figure 3.4   Interventions for the prevention of anaemia

much easier. Task definition and evaluation have in the past often been left out of health plans since they tend to fall in a no-man's-land between health planners and the trainers of health workers (see figure 3.5).

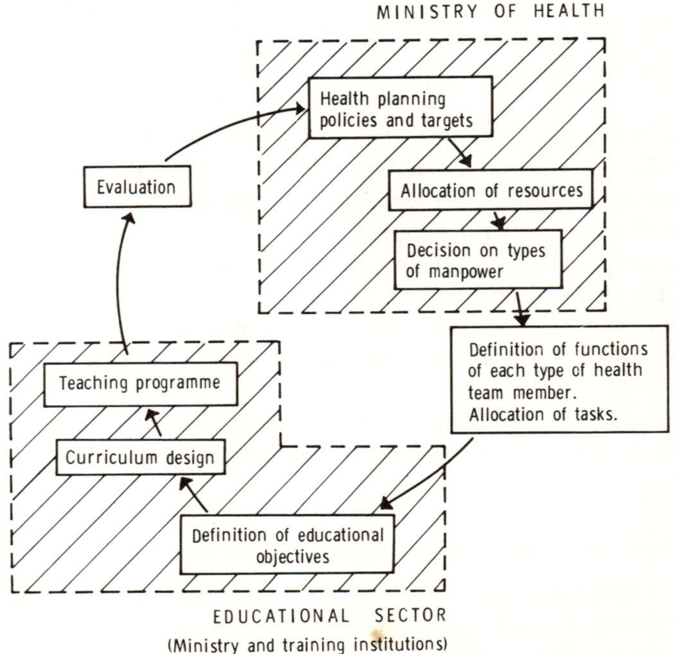

Figure 3.5   The usual no-man's-land of task definition and evaluation

In the past staffing was often decided by the population: health worker ratios, for example, the number of doctors or nurses or auxiliaries per unit of population. There were three major problems with this population ratio approach. The first problem is that of inequitable distribution. Although the National or Regional or District ratio of doctors to population may appear reasonable, it may hide gross differences in different parts of the district. Secondly, such a simplistic approach fails to take account of the accessibility of the health workers to the population. Few people travel for more than two hours (or 4–5 miles, 8 km) to a Health Centre or a sub-centre. It is not realistic to assume that Health Centres and similar facilities provide effective care beyond a distance of two hours' travel on foot. Thirdly, a population ratio approach may assume that mere provision of health manpower can provide good health. The tasks that the health workers perform may not be taken into account and the logistic support essential for efficient functioning may also get overlooked. For these reasons the 'functional approach' to health manpower planning has evolved.

The new 'functional' approach to district staffing (and health manpower planning) has as its starting point the three linked questions:

(i) What health tasks need to be done and can be done within the household and in the immediate community within a distance of one mile (1–2 km) from every home?

(ii) What back-up do these tasks require from the health team based at a health station 4–5 miles (8 km) away or within two hours' travelling distance?

(iii) What back-up does such a health team require from the District Health Team both at the community level and in the health station?

(vi) *Linking task setting and community involvement*

Community involvement in health care and action on determinants of ill health is essential. The community is the core of the District health strategy and all the health tasks and functions have a community component. The reasons for this are obvious. Local people are the greatest resource the District team has available. By working together the health care system will become part of the community's responsibility. It will not be seen merely as something remote run by the Ministry of Health. In drawing up a District Plan the challenge is to involve the local community in the process of task analysis and in the process of deciding who may be able to help with getting certain tasks done. In drawing up a District Plan, planners may either merely tell people to follow instructions so that they become dependent on instructions of what to do next. Alternatively, planners may work with the local community to try and tackle health problems together, and to take action on causes of ill health. This can encourage local initiative and new solutions to old problems (see figure 3.6).

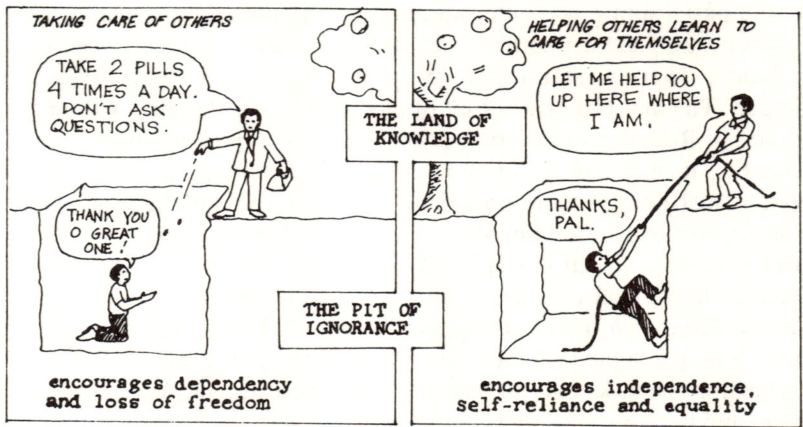

Figure 3.6   Encouraging self-reliance

(vii) *Matching needs to resources (allocating tasks to resources)*

Needs are often great, and resources limited, so another planning skill is allocating tasks to match available resources. The cycle is shown in figure 3.7 below.

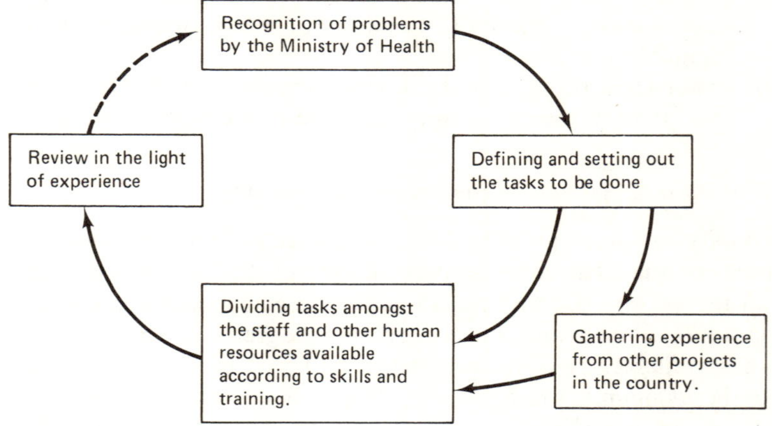

Figure 3.7   Matching needs to resources

(viii) *Liaison and team work*

Effective action on several of the more common health problems requires action in other related sectors besides health. Agricultural productivity is closely related to nutrition. Environmental sanitation is related to prevalence of worm infestations and diarrhoeal disease. Appropriate education is closely related to improved knowledge and understanding of disease causes, disease processes and how effective intervention can be done. Thus liaison between government departments is essential and barriers must be broken down for effective planning (see figure 3.8).

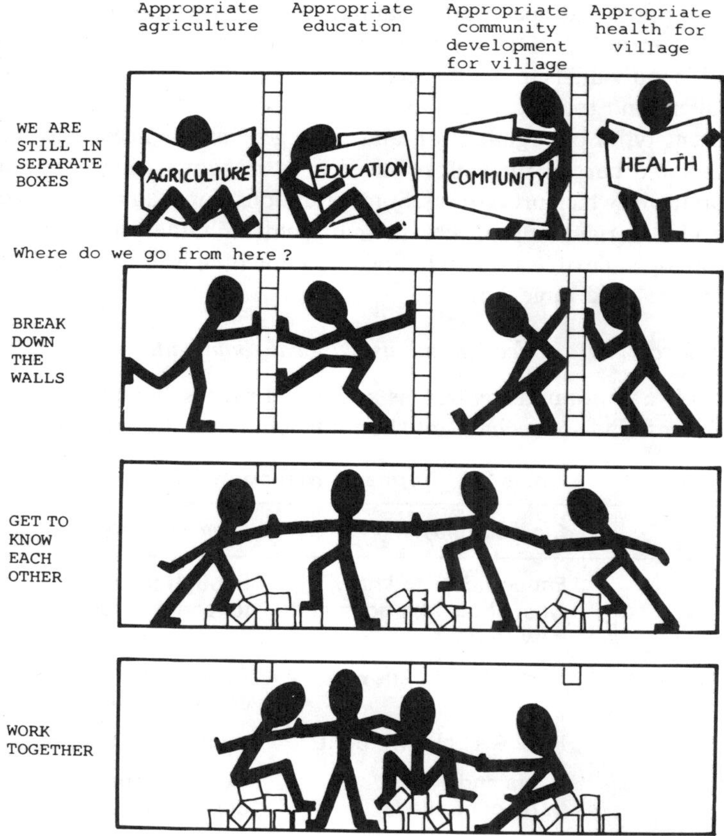

Figure 3.8   Liaison between government departments

(ix) *Learning from experience of projects, innovative approaches and so on (what goes well, what has gone wrong and what can be done)*

Some of the *relevant experiences* of how things can be done need to be specified using the experience of various projects. This procedure will then need to be complemented by specifying *also where things have gone wrong, and why, in the existing system*; unless these existing problems are overcome, and some solutions found, the same difficulties are likely to recur and be perpetuated into a new system. Much can be learnt from considering what has been successful (or not successful) in the past and why, and what has been found to work elsewhere. A number of new ideas so generated can be utilised for planning. Planners sometimes forget that theirs is never the first new approach to a problem.

(x) *Setting up a supportive organisation*

Logistic support and operational planning are other key issues recognised as essential in setting up a District Plan. An administrative set-up is needed which will enable individuals to work together, to make decisions regarding actions to be taken, and to supply support and supervision as needed.

Different types of organisation and management are needed in different situations and part of the skill required is to recognise what situations are appropriate for which procedures. Some situations (for example, emergencies) require closed rigid approaches in management. Other situations (most) require an open flexible approach if people's potential is to be fully developed (see chapter 4 and table 3.5).

(xi) *Feedback (data collection and use in local communities)*

Planning is a continuous as well as a learning process involving a series of cyclical steps, and so mechanisms should be built into the process which will

Table 3.5 **Types of management**

	Closed (rigid)	*Open (flexible)*
Data	Enough data to know what should be done and how to do it	Enough to start to learn by doing
Implementation	Using what is known	Avoid using and transmitting erroneous information
Evaluation	How well can we do it?	What is most important?
Changes	Errors and wrong: to be controlled	Expected and useful: opportunities to learn
Planning	Final plans before action	Tentative plan, constant revision during action
Nature of organisations	Unchangeable, internally stable, people come and go	People persist. Organisations constantly change
Authority	In manager with sufficient information to make decisions and get them implemented	In group with enough skills to make good decisions and to remove obstacles to their implementation

Source: Burkhalter, B. R. (c. 1978). *Modeling and simulation* vol. 5. Nutrition Planning Information Service, P.O. Box 8080, Ana Arbor, Michigan 48107, USA.

ensure that the information required locally, at health units and by the District team, is continually obtained. In the past many health workers have been asked to collect information which they then pass on to others for analysis and without any relevance to decision-making locally. The activity has therefore seemed a waste of time and many health workers have developed the bad habit of thinking that if they merely put in a certain number of hours they will have done their job adequately. *Jobs need to be geared to specific tasks instead of the hours spent at work.* The situation needs to be changed so that health workers can immediately assess for themselves the extent to which they have done a good day's or a good week's work. They have targets to aim for in the short and in the long term. With the involvement of local communities it is obvious that data collection, analysis and interpretation is needed at the very heart of the system, viz. the local community, so that immediate feedback of progress is available and decisions on new actions can be taken locally.

Feedback should also involve constructive criticism from those involved in putting the plan into action. Only by getting such criticism can a plan evolve and develop further. Local communities and local health facilities differ and each will need to work out how best to put the plan into action in their area.

Monitoring of progress also helps in getting feedback (see table 3.6).

Table 3.6 **Target setting and feedback mechanisms for five areas of a district plan**

Topic	Targets	Feedback
(a) Financial aspects	Budgeting in advance	Accurate accounting of what is spent
(b) Personnel	Detailed task centred job descriptions	Supervision to improve performance
(c) Supplies	Plan for the quantities required, their procurement and delivery	Monitor use and schedule maintenance
(d) Transport	Budget for mileage and maintenance	Maintain records on mileage and maintenance
(e) Community	Community diagnosis. Identify priority health problems	Community assessment of services, coverage, and utilisation

(xii) *Use of key procedures for training in primary health care*

Training is one of the most effective means of implementing a District Health Plan. It should be:

(a) *Focused on problems and tasks*

Training processes usefully include *problem orientation*, starting with a community diagnosis of priority health problems, developing approaches to the common health problems, trying to anticipate other difficulties and learning from such difficulties as are encountered on the job so that training continuously improves. In this way trainees will become equipped to deal with the type of problems they are likely to meet 'on the job'. Training then becomes *task-oriented*, focusing on the tasks to be done on the job when training is completed.

In the local community, training can be a way of mobilising local resources for health.

(b) *Focused on team work and multi-purpose workers*
Provision of health care relies on many people being able and prepared to work together. This is the common procedure in many societies. It needs to be reinforced. *Training for team work* may be helped by holding joint sessions for various topics. 'People do not learn much from what they are told. They learn from what they think, feel, discuss, see, and do together.'

Teams are needed at the local community level, the Health Station level, and in the District. Team members would have *joint responsibility* for the promotion of health and the prevention and treatment of disease in their area. They would have *overlapping roles* so that one team member can step in for another if someone is away or can cross-refer within the team to more specialised knowledge. All team members are expected to have a *general knowledge of the seven primary health care topics* (child health; maternity care; household environmental protection; community environmental health; community development; curative care and first aid; and communicable disease control). In addition, at each level (viz. the local community, the Health Station and the District), team members would have *specialist knowledge* in *Household Family Health, Community Environmental Health* or *Community Organisation for Development* (see figure 3.9).

In starting the training of local community workers it is probably unrealistic to try to train them all to do everything at once. They may not learn anything at all. Experience in different parts of the world indicates that for community health workers an on-going training programme with regular weekly, fortnightly or monthly sessions is more effective than longer courses held at infrequent intervals, or a one-off course.

There is a great need for multi-purpose workers. At the moment huge numbers of uni-purpose workers exist who cannot deal with the multiple causes of ill health. Further, there is minimal overlapping of roles amongst existing workers so if one worker is away, no work at all on that subject can be done. This is an uneconomic way of doing things. One answer to these problems is to aim for multi-purpose roles and teamwork.

The different teams are summarised in table 3.7 and figure 3.10. At the District level there is planning by a corporate team with specialist support when needed. At the Health Station level there is a multi-purpose team and at the local community level there are only multi-purpose workers.

Table 3.7 Team work and multi-purpose approaches

District level	Planning as a corporate team (Multi-purpose in content; Specialist in approach)
Health Station level	Multi-purpose team (with a few special areas of function)
Local Community level	Multi-purpose workers

Calculating degree of responsibility for each job to be done

The degree of the *responsibility* for care and for teamwork at each level needs to be analysed in order to work out the administrative and logistic support needed. The aim is to try to identify the exact work load and the components required to enable the specified tasks to be effectively and efficiently carried out.

Regular updating of training

Regular meetings and *regular refresher courses* are essential elements of in-service training. Health knowledge is changing so fast that everyone needs to try to keep up to date. Again, training cycles can be built into the plan.

Interchange between service and training

Another key process to maintain standards of training is the concept of *interchange between service and training responsibilities*. This means particularly exchange between administrative and clinical work at the Health Station, and training work with local community teams. It also means that any full-time District trainers (for initial PHC training) should rotate this responsibility with responsibility for running District services as part of the District Management team. There may also be similar exchanges between some hospital work and some Health Station work. In these ways training and service will remain closely linked together.

(xiii) *Specifying reasons and assumptions in planning*

In preparing guidelines on the tasks and training for a District Plan of Primary Health Care, the reasons for the decisions taken need to be specified so that people can understand how suggestions have come to be made. Wherever possible, assumptions need to be explained so that when the situation changes, the logical processes can easily be followed through again. The plan is a framework for further discussion and decisions at a local level.

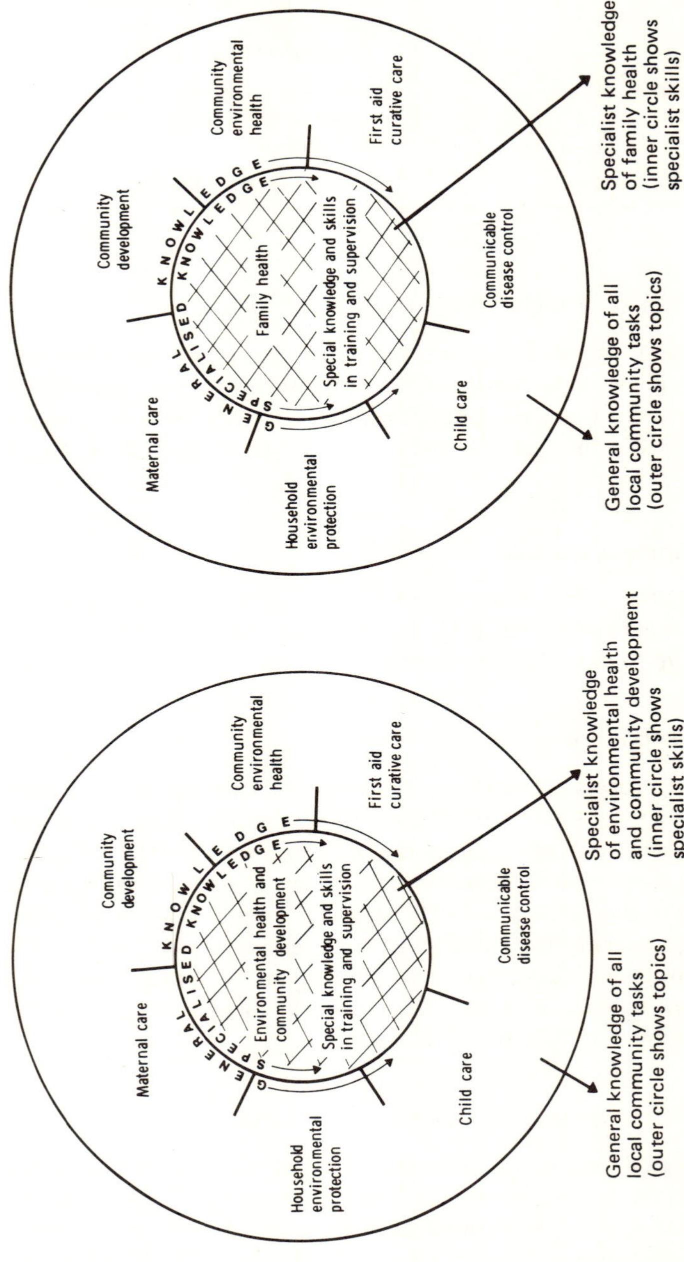

Figure 3.9   Distribution of general and specialist primary health care knowledge

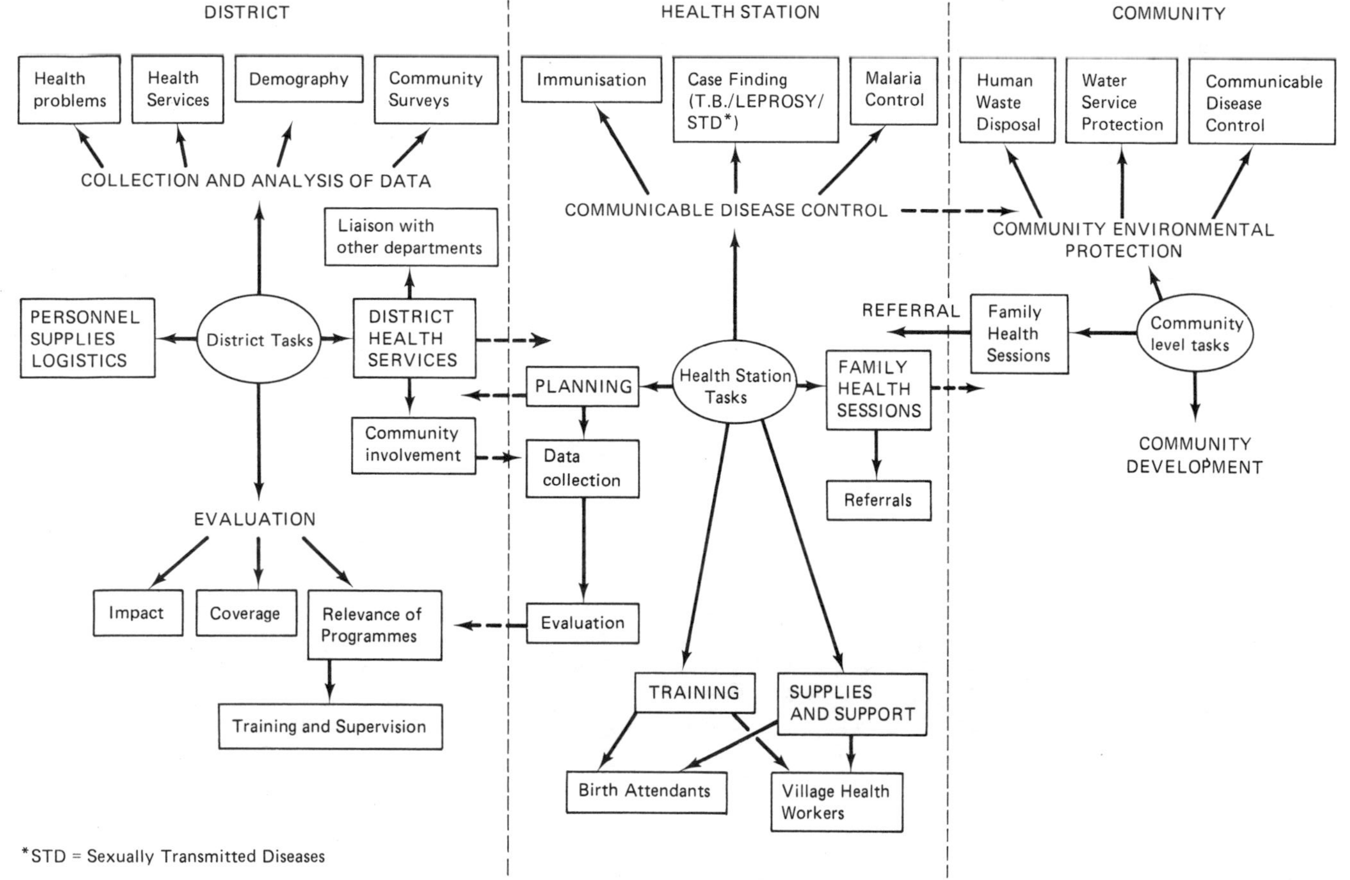

Figure 3.10   Teamwork and multi-purpose approaches

(xiv) *Holding reviews of progress*

This is frequently necessary with a complex task, in order to ascertain what proportion of the targets has been achieved. Often, further activity is dependent on achievement of earlier targets, and failure to do so in the apportioned time may delay further development of the health plan. The above key concepts of a District Health Plan are summarised in table 3.8.

Table 3.8   Key concepts behind a good district health plan

(i)   Priority health problems determine health service functions
(ii)   Health service functions determine accessibility needed
(iii) Health service functions also determine task definition and evaluation
(iv)   Health problems require action on causes of ill health, early intervention, and rehabilitation as well as care
(v)   Functions and task definition determine staffing (and Manpower planning)
(vi)   Linking of task setting and community involvement
(vii) Matching needs to resources (allocating tasks to resources available)
(viii) Liaison and team work
(ix)   Learning from local experience of projects, innovative approaches etc. what goes well, what has gone wrong, and what can be done
(x)   Setting up a supportive organisation
(xi)   Getting feedback (data collection and use in local communities)
(xii) Use of key procedures in training for primary health care
     (a) Training focused on problems and tasks
     (b) Training focused on team work and multi-purpose workers
     (c) Calculating the size of responsibility for each job to be done
     (d) Building in regular updating of training
     (e) Interchange between service and training
(xiii) Specifying reasons and assumptions in the plan

Examples of different elements of a district health plan

Four elements of making a District Health Plan are described in examples in this section. These are: (i) Recognising priority problems and relating them to health service functions and tasks; (ii) Planning and implementation whilst recognising what can go wrong; (iii) Planning training procedures and drawing on experience of what can go wrong; (iv) Calculating the degree of responsibility for each job to be done, how many staff are needed and what their requirements are likely to be. The example given is of maternity care.

(i) Recognising priority problems and relating them to health service functions and tasks at each level

The first step is to identify those problems which have priority on account of their prevalence, severity, community concern and the likelihood of response to management. The next step will be to decide on services that need to be provided in order to respond effectively to these problems. This is followed by agreeing the tasks which should be carried out for each service. Such a breakdown for maternity care is shown in table 3.9.

Table 3.9 Maternity service functions derived from priority maternal health problems

Priority maternal health problems	Contributing conditions or risk factors
(1) *Causes of maternal mortality*	
Ruptured uterus	disproportion*, malpresentation**, previous Caesarian section*, malposition**
Haemorrhage (mostly antepartum haemorrhage (APH), postpartum haemorrhage (PPH))	multiparity*, anaemia**, complicated delivery, abortions, placenta praevia
Puerperal sepsis	unhygienic procedures during delivery
Pre-eclamptic toxaemia	aetiology unknown – indications: high blood pressure, excessive weight gain**, clinical oedema, proteinuria**
(2) *Causes of neonatal and perinatal mortality and stillbirths*	
Birth injury	prolonged labour, abnormal presentation, disproportion*, etc.
Intrapartum asphyxia	toxaemia**, twins*, past and present malnutrition**,
Low birth weight	malaria**, primigravida*. Age over 40 and under 18*, previous stillbirth*
Tetanus	Unhygienic methods for cutting and tying the cord

* Can be detected at first antenatal visit
** Can be detected or prevented during antenatal period

Source: IDS Health Group, 1978. *Health needs and health services in rural Ghana.* Institute of Development Studies, University of Sussex, UK.

The next step is to recognise what is going wrong with existing maternity care services. Every society endeavours to care for mother and child. A District health organisation needs to build on what is already being done, and face difficulties where these are occurring. In a study of two Districts which examined all maternity care (amongst other types of care) provided at government and private maternity units, Health Centres and in outpatients at the District Hospital in Ghana a number of important shortcomings in the existing service were found. History taking of previous obstetric experience

was very poor (because it was often done by untrained personnel) and height
was rarely measured as an indicator of possible disproportion if pregnant
women were under 51 in. (145 cm). The 'risk concept' was not used except by a
few individuals, so there was little effective screening of high risk cases and
referral was not generally based on particular high risk categories. There were
shortages of tetanus immunisation, malaria prophylaxis and iron tablets.
There was little antenatal health education on home delivery (although many
mothers do deliver at home) nor on family planning. In both districts family
planning services were hardly available at all, in spite of considerable demand.
When mothers did need to be referred to the hospital in an emergency this was
extremely costly. Only one fifth of births were supervised by a trained
attendant, but for those that were supervised the standard of delivery care
seemed to be relatively good (see table 3.10).

Table 3.10 **Summary of existing maternal care problems in the district**

Data collection problems
History-taking problems
Need for height measurement
Need for tetanus immunisations, malaria prophylaxis and iron tablets
Need for effective screening and referral based on 'at risk' concept
Need for family planning and home delivery health education
Need for low cost emergency referral
Need for more coverage of family planning services
Need for more supervision of delivery by trained personnel

Source: IDS Health Group (1978).

The next step is to identify the defects and deficiencies in the existing
maternity care system. Such an exercise is essential because, until existing
difficulties are solved, there can be little point in attempting to extend the
services further into the community. All new ideas need to begin with the
retraining of existing staff.

Having recognised the health problems as well as the defects and deficiencies
in the existing health care system, and having specified the tasks to be done, the
next stage is to allocate the tasks to the available resources (see table 3.11). This
is also shown in figure 3.10 commencing with District Level tasks, those at the
level of the health stations and those to be carried out in the community.

(ii) *Planning implementation and recognising what can go wrong*

One crucial activity is to organise the logistic support and administrative
arrangements for the District health service. A check-list of basic logistical
support required will include the following:

(1) Existing record systems may need improvement. For example, the
    antenatal card or the Road to Health Chart may need a 'Risk' section
    and be action-oriented.

Table 3.11 **Maternal services: functions and allocation of tasks**

Functions of maternal services	*Tasks to be carried out*
Ensure normal delivery of a healthy baby and maintain mother in good health before, during and after delivery by:	Ensure (i) A minimum of 1 antenatal contact for all pregnant women (ii) An average of 3 antenatal contacts for 60% of pregnancies (iii) Where there is more than 1 antenatal contact, the first such contact to be in the first half of pregnancy
(1) *Antenatal care* for the purpose of: (i) diagnosis of mothers at risk of developing complications (ii) treatment of some complications and referral of others to facilities where more sophisticated management is provided (iii) prevention and treatment of diseases arising or exacerbated during pregnancy (e.g. anaemia, malaria) (iv) nutritional, health and family planning advice. (v) protection of the baby from tetanus.	*Antenatal care* (i) Take a history to identify the risk factors (ii) Refer those patients with risk factors (iii) Measure height and weight, fundal height and abdominal girth (iv) Check haemoglobin, blood pressure and urine. (v) Do clinical examination. Examine abdomen after 7/8 months. (vi) Give tetanus immunisation, malaria prophylaxis and iron and folic acid tablets (vii) Give advice on nutrition, checking on foetal movements, and on breast feeding
(2) *Supervision of deliveries*, for the purpose of: (i) ensuring aseptic techniques (ii) early detection and treatment of complications during delivery (iii) proper care of the newborn	*Delivery care* Supervise all births either directly or through trained village birth attendants (TBAs) (i) Monitor progress in labour using cervical dilatation charts to recognise complications early (ii) Look for signs of complications – foetal distress, bleeding, obstruction etc. (iii) Ensure hygienic techniques during labour (iv) Care of the newborn – ensure normal respiration, aseptic cutting and care of cord. Put the baby on mother's breast (v) Deliver placenta

Table 3.11   (*contd.*)

Functions of maternal services	Tasks to be carried out

(3) *Postnatal care*, for the purpose of
  (i) early diagnosis and treatment of complications in puerperium
  (ii) advising mother on newborn child care, nutrition, family planning
  (iii) provision of contraceptives
	Postnatal care
	Check condition of the mother. Look for fever, bleeding, tenderness of abdomen; check size of uterus; ensure adequate breast-feeding procedures. Advise on care of the baby. Give contraceptive advice.
	Family planning care
	  (i) Advise mothers and community on child-spacing
	  (ii) Provide contraceptives

(2) Requirements for transport need to be estimated and budgeted for.

(3) Equipment for the cold chain will also need to be similarly estimated and budgeted for.

(4) An essential drug list should be prepared for the district and circulated.

(5) A drug allocation system needs to be developed based on requirements rather than enlightened guesswork.

(6) A workable accounting and budgeting system needs to be developed.

(7) Laboratory and other services may need regular updating and maintenance.

People work more effectively if they have clear notions of their areas of responsibility and have been trained or given the opportunity to learn about the tasks they have to carry out. It is no use expecting doctors, nurses and other health personnel to come out of their training institutions knowing every detail of the tasks they are expected to perform. A considerable amount of training occurs on the job. There are other similar pitfalls which can affect the success of a District health programme. A check-list of management priorities to avoid pitfalls is given below:

(1) Clarify hospital responsibilities. Curative and surgical work has great attraction. If the staff assigned to hospital work are away, nurses and doctors from the District Health Team must not be moved to hospital duties.

(2) Clarify the work balance of the District Medical Officer (DMO). Up to half the time can be taken up by administration and the DMOs need to be prepared for it. Good and efficient administration is half the battle and if the DMO only does it sporadically and grudgingly, the District health programme will falter.

(3) Clarify the DMO's responsibilities for the staff, so that he should have

the authority to recruit, re-train, reprimand or recommend as the case
may be.

(4) Arrange for regular staff meetings. Job dissatisfaction is likely to arise
when health workers become isolated from their colleagues and feel
that they are shouldering all the responsibility alone. Several issues
may need airing to remove any doubts. Also, the nature of community
health activities is such that long-drawn-out and painstaking work and
negotiations are often needed, unlike curative work.

(5) Arrange for local collection, analysis and interpretation of data. Such
an exercise, carried out on a regular basis, helps the health team to
understand the progress being made towards the achievement of the
targets set in the health plan.

(6) Plan and arrange for staff training to match the tasks to be carried out
for providing health care in rural and peri-urban areas.

(7) Improve staff amenities and provide for more social meeting places.

(8) Rationalise pay differentials. It may not be possible to do anything
about salaries but perks can be rationalised. This applies especially to
private practice by the physicians and the specialists, which can be
restricted to a specified number of sessions per week.

(9) Many of the auxiliary staff may feel that they are in a career cul-de-sac
and cannot advance any more. Hence career development of the junior
staff requires thoughtful consideration. Encouraging upward mobility
creates a climate in which all the staff are working towards furthering
their knowledge and being rewarded for it.

(10) Improve the quality of care at the health stations through regular in-
service training, preparing a compendium of standardised procedures,
ensuring reliable supply of drugs and equipment, and of transport
when needed to reach remote communities.

What can go wrong with the health plan?

In trying to set up a new plan it is important to recognise the possible ways in
which things can go wrong. At the *Health Station Level* there are particular
traps to avoid. The main problem likely to arise at Level B is that inadequate
resources will be available to back up the work of the Health Station. In the
Primary Health Care system the Health Station staff are the key link between
the District team and local community workers. If they are to discharge this
responsibility effectively they need considerable support. If the current
problems of shortages or inappropriate training at Level B cannot be solved,
then it is unlikely that increasing the number of village health workers or
trained Traditional Birth Attendants is going to do any good.

Other problems are related to uncertainty concerning the involvement of the
community in Primary Health Care. Is it 'outreach' or 'involvement'? There
are several grades of participation beginning with nominating leaders to sit on

committees to a truly democratic dialogue with the community or its elected leaders. The latter approach is usually more successful in helping communities organise themselves for health as part of over-all rural and peri-urban development.

Procedures for liaison and co-ordination with agriculture, water resource development, education, social welfare, community development, and the district council, need to be worked out in detail. Special efforts are needed to forge links with extension and field workers who work closely with the local people.

Staff attitudes may cause difficulties at times. There may be unwillingness to work in rural areas; hospital work may be considered more prestigious; the primary aim may be to obtain a higher status in a chosen speciality rather than serve the people; the slant may be towards a high technology approach rather than making use of promotive techniques; and so on. Perhaps one cause of such attitudes is that in the average developing country two-thirds of the trainees come from the urban areas but two-thirds of the postings are to rural areas. Student selection procedures may need careful revision.

A number of things can go wrong at the *community level* in the working of a District Health Plan. In particular the following need careful consideration (see figures 3.11 and 3.12):

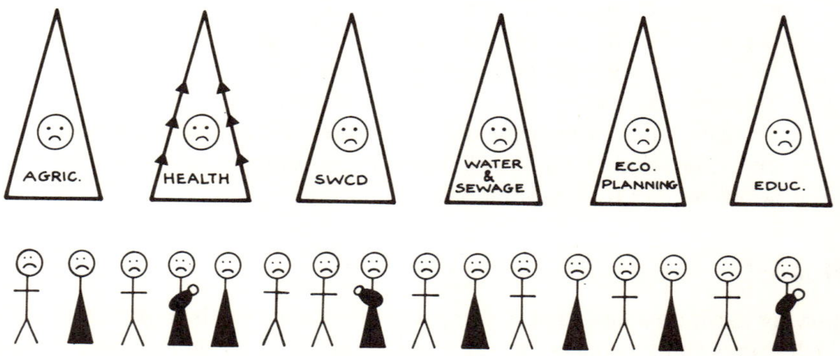

Figure 3.11   A 'top down' health care delivery system with a noticeable lack of co-ordination with other sectors, and little or no community involvement

(a) *Confusion between contribution and true involvement.* In the environmental or development activities people may be asked to contribute in cash or kind (material or labour). This is different from involvement, and is not a measure of participation. Involvement is to do with deciding about goals and tasks and working together to achieve this.

The alternative

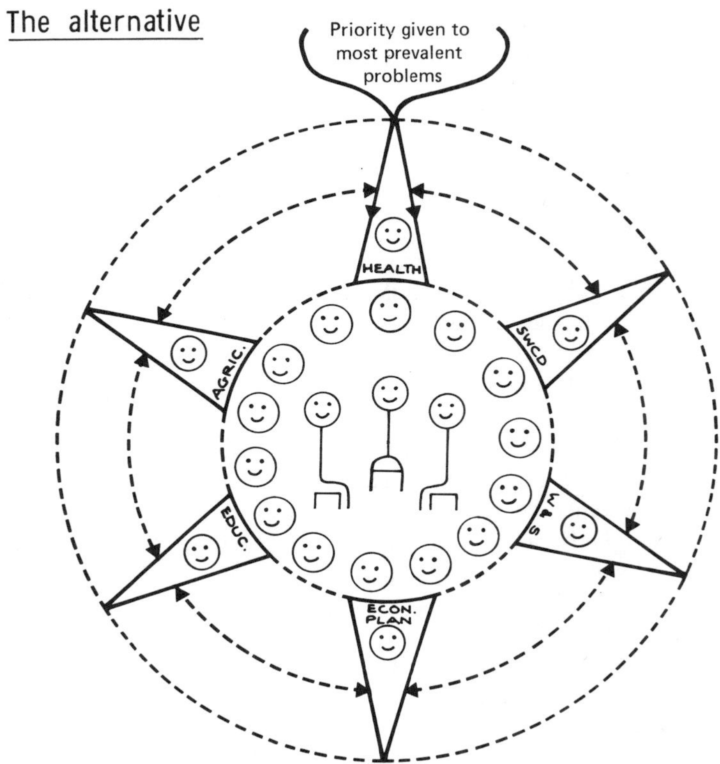

Figure 3.12   Community involvement in planning and implementation

(b) *Involvement of local people.* Although in theory participation of the people may be intended, in practice it may not take place. Community organisation and the formation of various social groups may be needed to achieve a high degree of awareness and sharing of responsibility.

(c) *Over-emphasis on structures.* Activities for generating community cohesion may get diverted into a programme of public works, or of amenities and ultimately end up as an administrator's programme.

(d) *Communities where contributions are too few or communal labour difficult to organise* may be neglected. These are usually the poorer communities where the struggle for survival is hard and leaves very little margin. Disappointments and frustrations may lead to the neglect of such communities.

(e) *Excessive decision-making by officials.* Instead of a framework of community health activities evolving out of community diagnosis, health care may be dispensed from above.

(f) *Continuing support may not be available.* It is necessary to maintain the enthusiasm generated at the commencement of the programme through regular feedback and involvement.

(iii) *Planning training procedures*

The main issue in setting up programmes of training in the District is to find teachers who like teaching and enjoy working with those they are going to teach. Topics need to be task-oriented and practical. At the end of each day synthesis and evaluation sessions may be arranged so that the trainers may assess whether a subject is too difficult or too threatening to the job expectations of the trainees.

At the District Level training requires not just the setting up of the initial training courses but also procedures for supervision as well as the continuing education of Health Station Level staff. This can be done through weekly or monthly meetings at the District centre, annual three-day visits to each Health Station, and an annual refresher course.

What can go wrong with District training? The staff-student ratio may be too low, there may be a lack of appropriate teaching material, trainees' experience may be ignored on the course, field training may contradict formal classes, and incentives for future work may be inadequate. There may be drop-outs of trainees and certain people may contradict the goals of the programme. There could be inadequate support of Level B workers by local community teams and inadequate governmental resources to maintain effective supervision. Insufficient time may be allowed for supervisory procedures and some staff, such as elderly dressers, may find it very difficult to learn. In all situations the need is to identify the problem precisely, to find out the reasons it has occurred, and to try and take action on the problem (see table 3.12).

Table 3.12 **Summary of guidelines for training family health workers at the level of the health station (Level B).**

1	Essential to have discussions with existing health unit personnel in devising course curricula.
2	Criteria for selection of staff could reflect the jobs expected from them, possibly using fictitious case studies to assess ability to solve common day-to-day problems.
3	Useful to have discussions with potential trainees prior to commencement of the training.
4	Use experience from other projects on selection and training for family health.
5	List 'tasks' to be covered in training.
6	Select teaching methods emphasising case studies and role play so that trainers learn by example those methods which are best for teaching local community workers.
7	Select relevant teaching material including texts and audio-visual aids.
8	Use the experiences of others regarding what can go wrong in training. Which solutions suggested are feasible for implementation locally?

Introductory sessions for training in the short and long term could usefully include case study descriptions of current local community work in the country. Training of the family health workers needs to be task-oriented so that they learn in turn how to plan a teaching and supervision programme for local community workers, how to keep records of local community supplies, how to liaise with others involved with local community workers (for example, other members of the Health Station team, referral midwives, agricultural field assistants, and so on) and how to evaluate local community training programmes. The teaching methods will need to make use of case studies and role playing so that during their studies the Health Station staff learn by personal experience the best methods for use in teaching Traditional Birth Attendants and other local community health workers (see tables 3.13 and 3.14).

Table 3.13 **Training the trainers of community health workers (Level A) needs to be task-oriented to include the following**

(a) Describing the tasks for community health workers and discussing plans with local chiefs, the village development committee and other representatives of the community.
(b) Identifying ways local communities could support community health workers (CHW).
(c) Describing criteria for the selection of CHWs so that local people could find suitable nominees.
(d) Seeing CHW nominees and discussing their job with them.
(e) Making an over-all plan for CHW training.
(f) Planning the training of CHWs, if necessary in several rounds.
(g) Planning on-going monthly supervision to cover one CHW task per month.
(h) Teaching CHWs by demonstration and role play.
(i) Keeping records of CHW training, supervision, supplies and problems.
(j) Organising supplies for CHW work.
(k) Liaising with other Health Station workers.
(l) Evaluating a CHW programme.

What can go wrong with the training of family health workers at health stations?

(1) The trainers may not know how to teach community and family health workers. They may not be interested in teaching them.
(2) Supervisors may not know what to do.
A suggested list of tasks for supervisors might include the following:

(a) Re-establish friendly rapport with community health workers.
(b) Discuss any problems they may have experienced in their practice or with referrals.
(c) Discuss any complications or deaths that have occurred since the last visit.

(d) Collect and record data on activities since the previous visit.
(e) Periodically evaluate the quality of work by observing the community health workers on their routine rounds.
(f) Replenish supplies (if this service is provided).
(g) Educate and update the knowledge of community health workers on one topic per month where necessary.
(h) Inform the community health worker of further activities such as refresher courses.

(3) Trainers may have difficulty preparing teaching material and record forms.
(4) Trainers may fail to form good relationships with nearby hospitals and Health Centres so that they are unprepared when asked to help with training or when they suddenly begin to receive referrals. Involvement of all participating institutions and sharing of information can help to avoid such difficulties.

Table 3.14 **Teaching methods need to emphasise *case studies* and *role playing* so that the trainers of CHWs learn by experience the methods that are best for teaching CHWs**

Examples
(a) Teaching methods might include accompanying trainees around the local community and asking them to spot 'nuisances', explaining what can be done by the community within its resources to prevent them.
(b) Another training procedure might be to arrange for trainees to meet relevant key personnel e.g. community development workers, agriculture extension officers, school teachers, etc.
(c) It would be essential to demonstrate simple construction skills for environmental improvement, perhaps at each of the Level A local communities.
(d) Organisation of communal labour might be taught through role playing to demonstrate what can go wrong.
(e) Each trainee might make a map of his own area, marking current environmental health problems and attaching a list of needs for community development.
(f) Demonstrations might be arranged at the trainee's own home and farm to show how food production can be improved.
(g) One session might be spent preparing a supervisory checklist from the CHW tasks.

Why do things go wrong with training?

The reasons for problems in the training programmes for health workers are many. Several of these problems stem from a lack of commitment to teaching found in many training institutions. In medical school, for example, teaching is often a secondary or tertiary activity after research and clinical work has been done. Secondly, lack of interest in teaching may arise from the very little time allocated to discussing teaching methods and organisation of training programmes in the medical and nursing curricula. Thirdly, promotion may depend on every other activity except teaching.

Another problem in training may be the separation of training from service delivery so that a great deal of the teaching tends to be theoretical. Without any first-hand field experience the students' first encounter with real problems is only after qualification.

Members of the health team who will have to work together are at present trained in separate institutions. There is a built-in separation of roles rather than attempts to hold people together through combined sessions. All these problems are often compounded by the large social gap between teachers and students, as well as between the different categories of health workers. This social barrier may exclude the possibility of interchange of ideas, problems and solutions.

The image portrayed by teachers will be very quickly adopted and emulated by the trainees. This is the so-called hidden curriculum. If teachers are only concerned with their status, think upon hospital curative work as the only health care that counts, are not innovative in their approach, and think that patients and students are annoying interferences in their daily life, then the trainees will also develop these attitudes.

(iv) *Calculating the degree of responsibility and the workload for each job to be done and how many staff are needed*

With some basic information about the community (for example, 20 per cent are children, the birth rate is 50 per 1000 population) it is possible to calculate the degree of responsibility held by each worker serving a particular population. An example is shown of the expected needs for child care in a community of 500 people, based on data from several studies (see table 3.15).

With such information, the degree of responsibility can also be calculated for the Health Station and District levels, for maternity care, adult sickness and environmental health as well as child care. The expected District responsibility for environmental health and community development is shown in table 3.16 in more detail, with a summary of responsibility for District level family health workers in table 3.17.

The need for a District Health Plan formulated through discussions and by consensus within the District Health Team is obvious for giving direction to the health activities within the District. Without such a direction towards defined objectives, health facilities will continue to perform routine tasks without making any tangible progress. But planning by itself is not enough. A true assessment of the health problems in the district is the first step towards successful planning. Attainable targets and objectives need to be defined and the health resources of the district need to be matched with the problems and the defined targets. The health personnel constitute the crucial part of the

Table 3.15 **Expected needs for child care in a community
of 500 people**

No. of children under 5 (20%)	= 100
No. of households	= 63
Weighing of 100 children monthly	= 1200 weighings per year
Family health sessions monthly	= 12 per year
Child sickness (5 contacts per child per year)	= 500 sick child visits per year
Child referral to Level B (20%)	= 100 referrals to level B per yr
Child referral to District care (10% from Level B)	= 10 referrals to level C per yr
Child adms. to District Hospital (25% of referrals to Level C)	= 2–3 children per yr hospitalised
Meetings with other local comm. workers (monthly)	= 12 per year
Meetings with Level B staff visiting Level A (weekly)	= 52 per year
Meetings at Health Stations (monthly)	= 12 per year
Meetings (bi-monthly) at Level A for home visits etc.	= 6 per year

Table 3.16 **Tasks in the district for environmental health and
community development**

(i)   *Tasks*

For 20 health station teams each with 10 local community teams, total
200 local communities, maximum 100 000 population, if *all* tasks were to
be done, the district community health responsibility needed would
include:

200–400	water sources	(1–2 per 500 people)
200	public latrines	(1 drophole per 40 people, 2500 dropholes)
200–400	refuse dumps	(1–2 per 500 people)
200	market places	(1 per 500 people)
200–400	chop bars	(1–2 per 500 people)
200–400	school food traders	(1–2 per 500 people)
200–400	drinking bars	(1–2 per 500 people)
? 200	community farms and gardens	(1 per 500 people)
200	community day care facilities	(1 per 500 people)
200	local income earning activities	(1 per 500 people)
1200	community labour activities	(6 per local community per year, minimum)
200	community projects needing district advice once or twice	(2 per local community per year, minimum)

Table 3.16 *(contd.)*

To be estimated: CDC incidence, spraying, mass campaigns and individual care needed.

TOTAL 3400–4400 ongoing activities in all

However, if most Health Workers were doing only the top priority tasks, only some of these projects might be in operation.

(ii) *Area: 25 mile (40.2 km) radius, 1963 sq. miles (5076 sq. km)*
The area covered by the district team would be not more than a radius of 25 miles (40.2 km) from the district base (to enable a round trip of 50 miles (80.4 km) maximum). The maximum total area would be 1963 sq. miles (5076 sq. km).

(iii) *Population: 100 000 people maximum per district team*
It is assumed that one district team could be responsible for a maximum population of 100 000 people (see workload below).

With the distribution of responsibility for 100 000 population into 20 health station teams (1 team per 5000 people) and 200 local community teams (1 team per 500 people) the expected community health responsibility and workload would be as follows (if the distribution of the responsibility for the 100 000 people was different some aspects of the workload would of course differ too).

(iv) *Expected local community Level A workers per district team (100 000 people)*
(In low density areas one Level A worker might be providing top priority tasks only for all three areas, community health, maternal care and child care).
    200 community health organisers (1 CHW for top priority tasks for 500 people)

200 retrained TBAS   which the district MCH supervisor will
200 household family   need to supervise from the health
   health workers   station.

Expected health station (Level B) MCH workers per district team for 100 000 people)
20 health station MCH workers.

CDC = Communicable Diseases Control
CHW = Community Health Worker
MCH = Mother and Child Health
TBA = Traditional Birth Attendant (also Trained BA)

Table 3.17 **Summary of responsibility for district family health specialists serving a population of 100 000 people**

No. of family health workers	= 200 (1 per 500 people)
No. of traditional birth attendants	= 200 (1 per 500 people)
No. of community health workers (for monthly supervision)	= 200 (1 per 500 people)

Table 3.17   *(contd.)*

Maternal care

No. of households	=	12 500
Expected number of births	=	5 000 per year
Deliveries by TBAs (?60% births)	=	3 000 per year
Deliveries by Health Station staff (30% births)	=	1 500 per year
Standard antenatal contacts for TBAs (3 per pregnancy)	=	15 000 per year
Standard antenatal contacts for Level B staff (2 per pregnancy)	=	10 000 per year
At risk antenatal contacts for Level B staff (20% pregnancies) 3 extra contacts	=	9 000 per year
Emergency in labour referral to Level C (10% pregnancies)	=	500 per year
Postnatal care by TBAs (3 per birth)	=	15 000 per year
Postnatal care at the Health Station	=	to be estimated

Child care in the district (per 100 000 population)

Number of children under 5 (20%)	=	20 000
Number of households registered	=	12 500
Weighing of 20 000 children monthly	=	240 000 weighings per year
Family health sessions monthly (200 communities)	=	2 400 per year
Child sickness at Level A (5 contacts per child per year)	=	100 000 sick child contacts
Child sickness referred to Level B (20%)	=	20 000 sick child events referred per year
Child sickness referral to Level C (District) (10% of those at Level B)	=	2 000 per year
Child admission to District Hospital (25% of those referred to the District level)	=	500 per year

Household health care

Average household size = 8 people
Number of households = 12 500

12 500 kitchens and kitchen hazards
12 500 water storage systems
12 500 household faeces disposal methods
12 500 waste water seepaways
12 500 food storage methods and vermin hazards
12 500 sleeping places potentially hazardous for spreading tuberculosis and other communicable diseases
(??) incidence of communicable diseases

Adult sickness care per 100 000 population in district

Number of adults over 15 (55% population)	=	55 000
Number of households	=	12 500

Table 3.17   (*contd.*)

Family health sessions monthly	=	240 per year
Adult sickness (2 contacts per adult per year)	=	110 000 per year
Adult referral to Level B staff (20%)		
(to family health session if possible)	=	22 000 per year
Adult referral to Level C (District care)		
(10% of those referred to Level B)	=	2 200 per year
Adult admission to District Hospital		
(25% of those referred to Level C)	=	550 per year

health resources of the District. Their training, deployment and technical as well as administrative support at all levels is a major challenge in health management. In the absence of such back-up and support of the workers even the most carefully designed plans cannot succeed. Hence the importance of building up an effective health organisation which will ensure that the right personnel are deployed at the right level and regularly receive the material and equipment to deal with the tasks set for that level. The key concepts and principles of evolving an effective District health organisation are considered in the next chapter.

FURTHER READING

Gish, O. *Guidelines for Health Planners. The Planning and Management of Health Services in Developing Countries*, TRI-MED, London, 1977.

Ministry of Public Health, *Lampang Health Development Project*, vols I to V, Ministry of Public Health, Thailand, 1981.

World Health Organization, *Formulating Strategies for Health for All by the Year 2000*, WHO, Geneva, 1979.

4 Building the Health Organisation in the District

Probably the most important instrument available to a District Medical Officer (DMO) in charge of the 'District Health Team' for implementing a Primary Health Care Plan is the organisation of the team. One of the marks of the DMO as a successful manager is the ability to visualise the health personnel and other resources of the district as an organisation, disposed in the most effective way throughout the District to combat its health problems. Just as the health plan gives a clear analysis of the health needs of the District and the most effective way of meeting them, so the organisation is the means of translating the objectives of the health plan into practical action. Where there is good organisation the health personnel are able to work to their full potential, and the many different aspects of health care carried out by different people can be integrated for maximum effect. It is only within a sound organisation that good management can take place. There are many examples of individuals whose work has been unsatisfactory but which has improved enormously when they have either been moved to a different organisation or to another part of the same organisation, or the organisation itself has been changed in some way. What has been at fault is not the individual, but the organisation.

FORMAL AND INFORMAL ORGANISATION

A distinction can be made between a 'formal' and an 'informal' organisation, each of which has advantages in certain situations.

A formal organisation is often described by means of an 'organisation chart' such as those which appear in figures 4.1 and 4.2.

Among the advantages of formal organisation charts are that they:

(a) define broad areas of job responsibility;
(b) provide a basis for writing job descriptions;

(c) indicate channels of communication;
(d) clarify relationships between people;
(e) avoid complications caused by overlapping of functions.

Probably their most useful function is in the thought process the manager must go through in drawing up the chart in the first place. It requires thinking about who actually is in the organisation, what work they do, and whom they relate to.

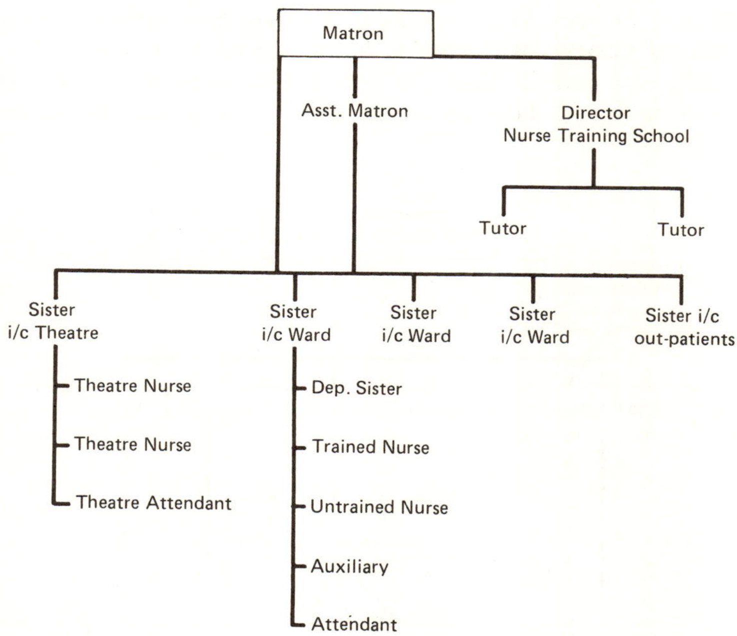

Figure 4.1   An organisation with relatively few different types of activity

Figure 4.2 shows the managerial and communications structure of a Primary Health Care organisation. Level B (the Health Centre) teams form the crucial Middle Management level between the local community workers and the District Health Management Team. The position on the chart of the Town or Village Development Committee indicates its important managerial position in relation to Level B staff. These staff are technical advisers to the Town or Village Development Committee. The local community workers come directly under the management of this committee for everything except technical matters like selection, discipline, and so on.

AN ORGANISATION AS A SKILL PYRAMID

It helps to look upon a District Health Organisation as a 'skill pyramid', as in figure 4.3. Such an attitude recognises that there are only a few health workers with particular medical skills and knowledge, and that their function is to diffuse their expertise throughout the community by means of the health organisation. At the same time, there is a great deal of local knowledge and information about the community and its health which needs to come into the organisation and to be used for planning or for the organisation of services. The effective District Medical Officer and his Management Team are concerned to achieve and sustain an organisation in which skill and responsibility are pushed 'down' the organisation as far as possible, and in which information can flow 'up' the organisation as quickly as possible.

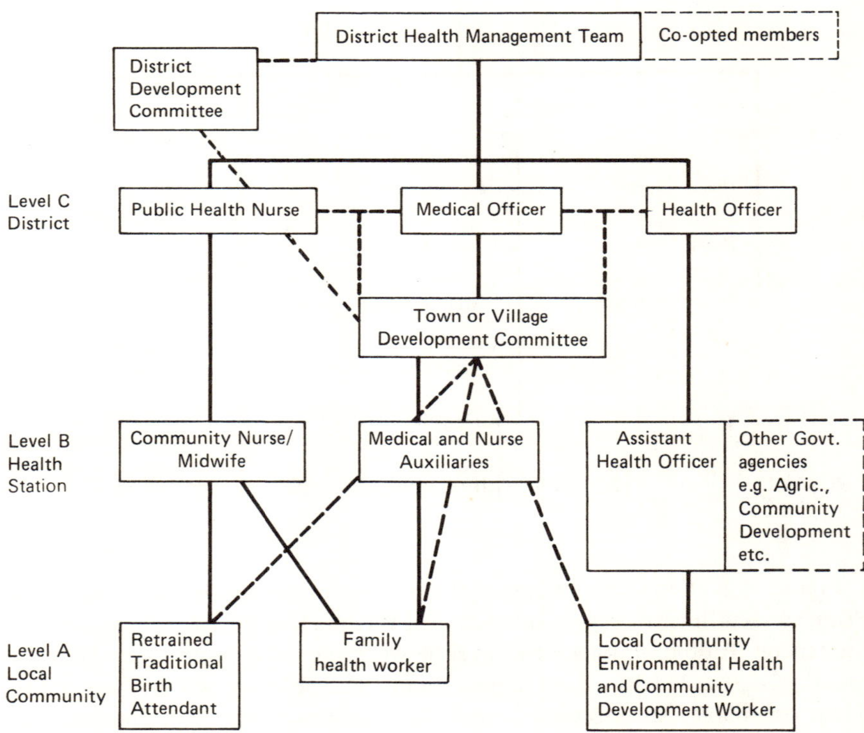

Figure 4.2   Organisational structure of a primary health care system showing managerial and communications structure (adapted from Ministry of Health, Ghana, 1980)

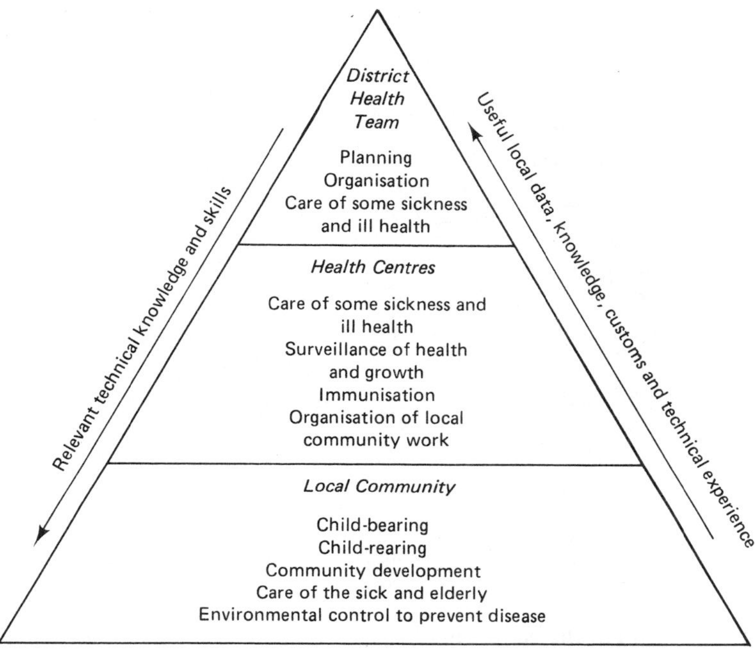

Figure 4.3   An organisation as a skill pyramid

AN ORGANISATION AS A NETWORK OF INDIVIDUALS

The District Health Organisation can also be considered as a *network* of individuals, groups and agencies. The function of the District Management Team is to develop and extend the network rather like a spider's web, to encompass and knit together all those who contribute to the improvement of the health of the population.

Figure 4.4 is an example of a 'network' for a District Health Team. It can be a useful exercise for any DMO to map out his or her 'network of relationships'. It is useful to indicate which of the relationships are most important so far as achieving the current objectives is concerned, and what the current state of relationships is to different people. This can then show which relationships need to be developed more so that any necessary improvements can be made. It is also useful to look at relationships in terms of expectations — both what you are expecting other people to do for you and what they expect of the health team. In considering these expectations, and where necessary making changes through discussion and agreement with the people concerned, the District Health Team can do much to direct the attention of the

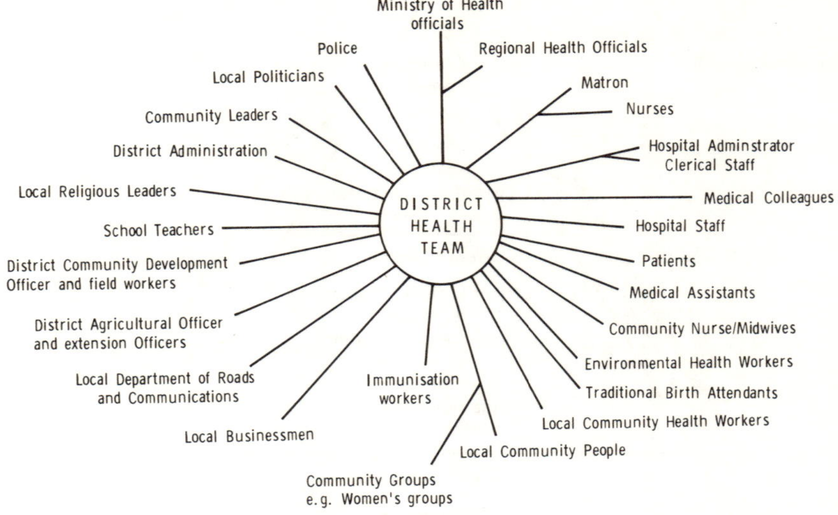

Figure 4.4　　　　　The network of relationships for the district health team

organisation and of the people in it to the matters of most importance, besides thinking seriously about the team's priorities in the most efficient use of time.

AN ORGANISATION AS A SYSTEM OR SERIES OF SYSTEMS FOR GETTING THINGS DONE

We can think of an organisation as a system which is a collection of inputs, processes and outputs. In a health organisation a *simple common integrated system is needed* to bring together a number of separate systems concerned with the movement of drugs, supplies, information, people, referrals and cash. This integrated system will need to flow according to need daily, weekly and monthly between the local community, the middle level and the District centre. Some examples of systems and the features of a good system are considered in table 4.1.

Two major 'systems' can be distinguished which influence primary health care. These are the 'local traditional system' of decision-making and organisation and the 'imported bureaucratic management' approach.

Many of the ideas of management in the bureaucratic system have evolved in relation to large organisations in industrial and commercial enterprises and public services, particularly in North America and Europe. This approach to management developed alongside rapid economic growth in those countries, and has been a basis for the organisation of government and state services.

This kind of bureaucratic management is best exemplified in the large international organisations like the multi-national companies, or in international agencies. For carrying out certain kinds of tasks on a large scale such a system is ideal.

The best example in the health field is probably the systematic eradication of smallpox which was effectively planned, organised and carried out on a global scale with the backing of the World Health Organization. When the local health organisation receives funds from government sources and is part of a National health strategy, then many of the techniques of this type of management will be needed.

Table 4.1 **Examples of systems and features of a good system**

Examples of systems	*Features of a good system*	
Budgeting	1	Regulation of inputs and outputs.
Supplies	2	Makes complexity simple.
Prescribing	3	Eliminates oversight.
Referral	4	Relevant.
Maintenance	5	Wide applicability.
Transport	6	Comprehensive.
Payment	7	Integrated with others
Supervision	8	Regularly reviewed.
Planning	9	Simple to understand.
Information	10	Attractive to use.
Evaluation		
Recruitment		
Training		
Accounting		
Audit		

Before such a systematic approach came to be developed, however, there were other ways of getting things done. The traditional system still exists in many communities. Although it may appear to differ from place to place there are often common features in this type of organisation in many societies. Features include respect for the views of elders in the community, decision-making only after lengthy discussion by the whole community, formal means of appointing leaders often on a hereditary basis, recognised ways of providing help for members of the community in need, and punishment for those who transgress the community's legal and moral code. In developing Primary Health Care in any community it is folly to ignore the way in which the community organises itself, and this is particularly so in the more traditional outlying rural village communities.

Successful organisation of Primary Health Care therefore requires the ability to understand and work within the two systems, viz. the modern bureaucratic form of management, and the traditional. Diagramatically (see figure 4.5) the two systems can be represented as pyramids: the modern management system as an inverted pyramid with its weight and strength in national and governmental policies, plans, resources and organisation which are translated through the District Health Organisation to create an impact on people living in their rural, peri-urban, and urban communities; the traditional system as a pyramid on its base, with its weight and strength widely distributed in local communities but also having an impact in the life and organisation of the country at District, Provincial and National levels.

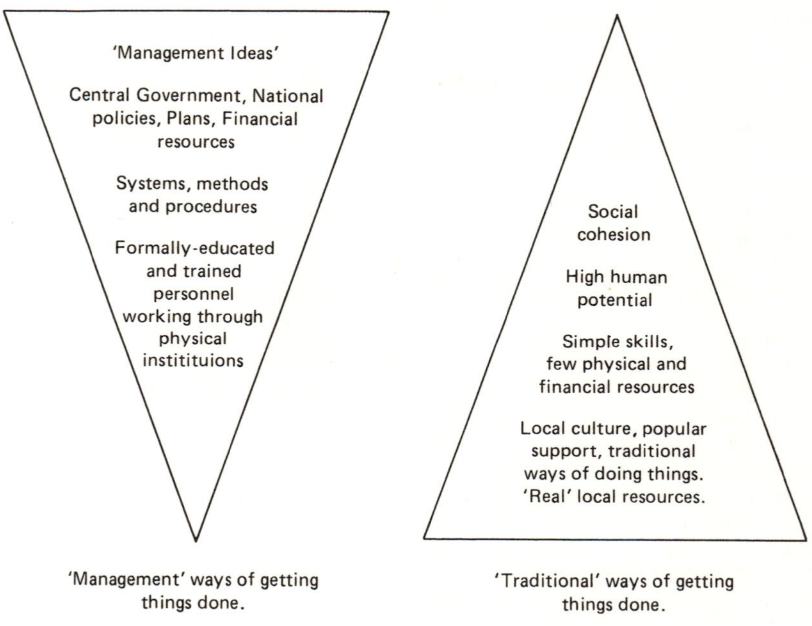

Figure 4.5   'Management' and 'traditional' ways of getting things done

If we next consider a rural health care system in terms of Level A (local community health workers), Level B (Health Centre serving a number of villages), and Level C (District, including hospital services) linked to the Provincial or Regional and National levels of health care and then superimpose our 'models' of 'management' and 'traditional' systems, we get an interesting result (see figure 4.6). The point at which the two systems coincide to the greatest extent is at Level C, the level of the District Health Team. The District Health Team becomes the key point in the over-all health system for integrating the concept of 'management' and 'traditional' systems. This means that the District Health Team should have:

(a) a good *knowledge* of both systems;

TYPICAL ACTIVITIES	TYPICAL INSTITUTIONS	LEVEL
Interchange of ideas Strategic planning International approach	World Health Organisations International Aid Agencies Multi-National Drug Companies	INTERNATIONAL
National planning and priorities High professional training (Teaching hospitals)	Ministry of Health Institute of Traditional Medicine Council of Chiefs	NATIONAL
Provincial planning Professional training	Provincial/Regional Medical/Environmental Health Officials	PROVINCIAL
Organisations and running of District services Support to locally-based health activities	District Health Team District Hospital Paramount Chieftaincies Renowned traditional healers	LEVEL "C"
Practical and simply organised preventive and curative health services	Health Stations Local Chiefs Local traditional healers	LEVEL "B"
Healthy living as a normal part of village life Basic preventive and first aid services	Local Community Council Local Health Workers Traditional Birth Attendants	LEVEL "A"

Figure 4.6   Intersection of 'traditional' and 'management' systems

(b) a good *understanding* of the strengths and weaknesses of both systems;
(c) the ability to work within both systems so that the strengths of each can be brought together to produce the most effective health system;
(d) the ability to *interpret* to those who are predominantly involved in one system, the contribution which the other system can make towards solving their problems;
(e) the ability to be *creative* in adapting and devising new systems which take into account the advantages of both.

The traditional system is already being influenced by the external system. The challenge is now to enable the traditional system to take from the external system those things which are genuinely useful in a way which does not destroy its own effectiveness, culture and values. In the process the external system may be influenced by what is good in the internal traditional approach.

SOME KEY PRINCIPLES IN AN EFFECTIVE ORGANISATION

Much is written about 'Principles of Organisation'. Table 4.2 lists ten Principles of Organisation. The District Health Team will probably be most concerned with *co-ordination*, making sure that the different parts of the organisation (for example, local community workers, Health Centre staff) do not work in isolation but work together towards a common goal. It must be clear also where authority and responsibility lie for any individual at any one time.

Take the example of a nurse in training who accompanies the epidemic emergency team to gain practical experience as part of her training programme. The nature of her relationship to the team leader, to the nurse on the epidemic emergency team, to her Nurse Tutor, and so on needs to be clear if she is not to be put into the position of having to take contradictory instructions from different people, or of not knowing whom to approach with a particular problem.

Table 4.2 **Some principles of effective organisation**

1 *The Principle of Co-ordination*
   The purpose of organisation is to facilitate co-ordination; unity of effort.
2 *The Span of Control*
   No person should supervise more than five, or at the most, six, direct subordinates whose work interlocks.
3 *Definitions and job descriptions*
   The content of each position, both the duties involved, the authority and responsibility contemplated and the relationships with other positions, should be clearly defined in writing and published to all concerned.
4 *The Principle of Continuity*
   Re-organisation is a continuous process; in every undertaking specific provision needs to be made for it.
5 *The over-all Objective*
   Every organisation and every part of the organisation needs to be an expression of the over-all aim of the undertaking. Otherwise it is meaningless and therefore redundant.
6 *Authority*
   In every organised group the supreme authority must rest somewhere. There should be a clear line of authority from the supreme authority to every individual in the group.
7 *Responsibility*
   A superior is always completely responsible for the acts of a junior worker.
8 *Correspondence of responsibility and authority*
   In every position the responsibility and the authority should correspond.
9 *The Principle of Balance*
   It is essential that the various units of an organisation should be kept in balance.
10 *Specialisation*
   The activities of every member of any large organised group can sometimes usefully be confined to the performance of a single function.

Span of Control is also important where there are large numbers of scattered local community health workers. To give them adequate supervision and support may entail grouping them under the supervision of perhaps a community nurse midwife or a medical assistant based at a rural health centre. If the span of control is too large, for example, with very large groups to supervise, people get neglected. If too small, there is wasteful duplication. *Job*

Descriptions are a well-established way of dealing with the principle of definition, to ensure that the duties, authority and relationships of each post are clearly defined within the organisation. Table 1.14 (The PHW profile) in chapter 1 and table 4.3 below are broad statements of the job requirements for two jobs, a Primary Health worker, and a medical assistant, prepared as guides for those working in the rural health field.

Table 4.3 **Job description of a medical assistant**

Organisational Relationships

Functions

Administration	. Administration of the Health Centre.
	. Supervision and co-ordination of the team of health workers.
	. Supervision of satellite health posts and dispensaries.
	. Production of quarterly reports to District or Regional MOH.
Curative	. Diagnosis and treatment of illness (or referral).
Community Work	. Implement Health and Research Community Programme.
	. Encourage members of community to be involved in health programmes.
	. Convene team members to co-ordinate activities.
	. Participate in village development programmes.
	. Collect and report data – sociological/epidemiological, morbidity/mortality.
	. Give support to VHWs – regularly in their villages – through training activities in the health centre and elsewhere.

Source: Health Auxiliaries and the Health Team. Eds Muriel Skeet and Katharine Elliott, p. 156.

These are general descriptions but it is important always to make the job description fit specific situations. A good way of doing this is through discussions aimed at clarifying exactly what a job holder is trying to achieve in his or her work. There are dangers in job descriptions which are too detailed and rigid. Any job is likely to change in the course of time, and different people are likely to do the same job in somewhat different ways depending on the background, interests, experience and so on of those individuals. One way of avoiding rigid job descriptions is to *put an emphasis on the 'outcome' of a job* or *what* has to be achieved in a person's work, rather than a detailed specification of *how* that work is to be done (see figure 4.7).

The principle of *continuity* is an important one. As conditions change, staff come and go, new ideas are introduced and there will be a need to change and improve the organisation. Major organisational change usually causes upset to the people concerned, but by being in close touch with the organisation and

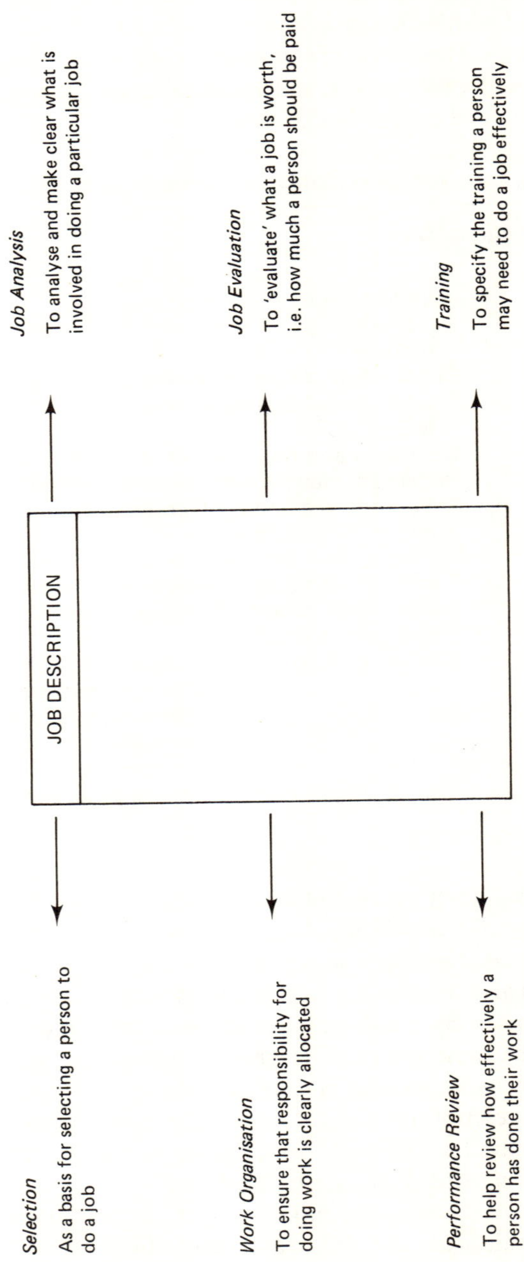

Figure 4.7   Uses of a job description

anticipating and making changes as they become necessary, senior managers can often avoid the need for more radical changes later.

THE KEY ELEMENTS OF AN EFFECTIVE ORGANISATION

With a little skill and some experience it is not difficult to view an organisation and detect where changes need to be made. The good manager identifies malfunctioning, diagnoses particular problems and prescribes corrective action. But it is then necessary to get the organisation to take the corrective action which may be the most difficult part of the process. As with health, so also with organisations; prevention is often better than cure. The effective manager will constantly be taking action to prevent the organisation getting into major difficulties. There are a number of elements to an effective district health organisation, as shown in table 4.4.

Table 4.4 **Four key components of an effective district health organisation**

Analysis of problems
Development of ideas to tackle them (plan)
Administration of supplies, equipment, transport, personnel
Leadership of people

Each of these four topics has to be organised well (see figure 4.8). The process of setting tasks which needs to be developed as a result of problem analysis has already been described.

The planning process then becomes the development of a course of action. It entails the gathering of data, identifying the causes of problems and developing alternative solutions. This needs setting priorities and the development of policies. It also needs resource allocation through budgeting, then programming, formulating strategic plans on how and when to achieve goals, specification of the end results expected (objectives) and targets to establish where the present course of action will lead.

The administrative organisation is simply the arrangement of work to accomplish the objectives effectively. It requires definition of the skills needed for the tasks to be performed in each position in the organisation. Each needs a specification of scope, of responsibility and authority and a defined relationship to others.

People recruited into the organisation need to be provided with a setting in which they can work purposefully and effectively towards the objectives. Finding the right people is clearly crucial. After selection they need to be familiarised with the situation, trained, and then helped to improve their knowledge, attitudes and skills. Their responsibilities and accountability need

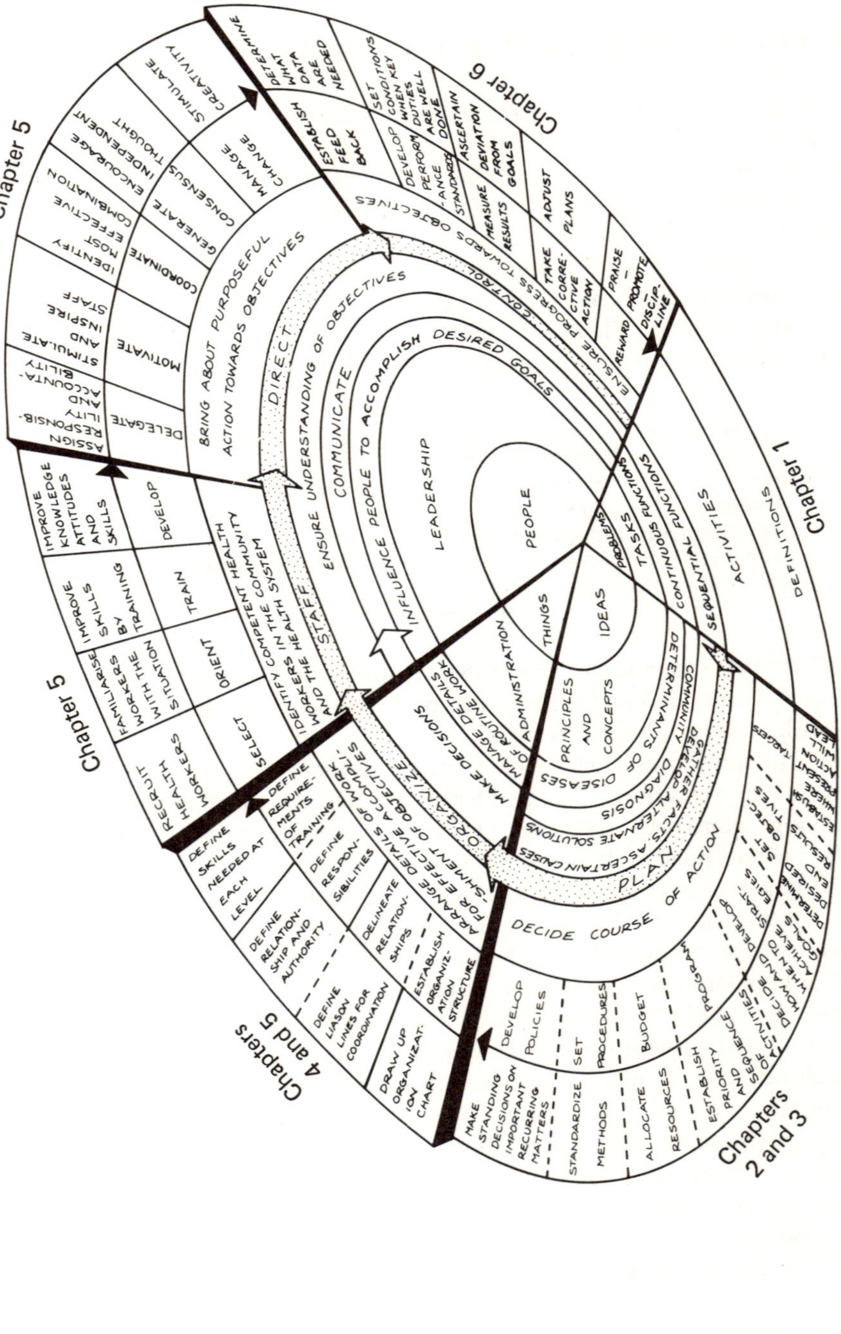

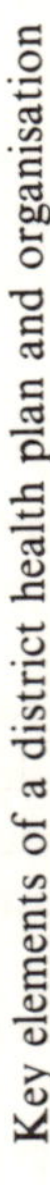

Figure 4.8   Key elements of a district health plan and organisation

careful defining if delegation and co-ordination is to work. Independent thought needs to be fostered and people inspired or encouraged to think for themselves. Differences in opinion need to be managed and conflict resolved. Change needs to be managed too, through stimulating creativity and innovation in achieving goals. Control is needed to make sure that progress is made towards the objectives of the plan. A reporting system is needed so that people know what data are required, and how and when to produce them. Performance standards may be set which indicate what specific conditions exist when key duties are well done. Results can then be measured from both these sources to see any deviation from standards, and corrective action can be taken to adjust plans and standards if needed. Discipline may be necessary at times, but reward, praise and remuneration are just as important as means of control and incentive.

What it means to manage a district health organisation

In order to work efficiently a rural health district has to be well organised and run. The District Health Team and the District Medical Officer need to appreciate that their work is to a large extent managerial. Unfortunately in the past doctors and other health workers have not been trained to think of themselves as managers but rather tended to take their teachers, the hospital consultants, as models. So we need to try and answer the question: what does it mean to be a manager? This is shown in table 4.5.

Table 4.5 **What does it mean to be a manager?**

1	Seeing the whole picture (i.e. beyond the hospital, and the entire district as their area of responsibility).
2	Good personal motivation.
3	Recognising contributions which further the aims of the organisation.
4	Effective use of time.
5	Standards of performance.
6	Clear objectives.
7	Planning the future while managing the present.
8	Organising and allocating resources.
9	Decision-making.
10	Delegating, motivating and developing other people.
11	Developing and maintaining systems.
12	Reviewing and evaluating.
13	Being an agent of change.

(1) *Seeing the whole picture*

The problem of many professionals and specialists is that they see things in the light of their own expertise and do not find it easy to appreciate the point of view of others. But the manager must have a broader view. In fact, a manager needs to be a professional 'non-specialist'. All the advice available from specialists is taken, but it must always be put into the context of the whole situation. District Health Managers need to be able to see the whole of the Health District, its needs and problems, as it were, from without rather than from within.

(2) *Good personal motivation*

The attitude of a manager sooner or later affects the whole organisation. If the manager is apathetic, not interested and disillusioned about work, then these attitudes will spread to others, and even keen and enthusiastic workers will stop trying, or look for other ways of channelling their energies. So managers need to be sure that their job is worth doing, and that they are totally committed to it.

(3) *Recognising contributions to the aims of the organisation*

The good manager has a very clear idea of what contribution good management can make to the total success of the work of the Health District. From time to time he will look up from his work and ask 'What is the best contribution I can make to the goals of this Health District?'. At the same time, the manager asks about other workers in the district 'What is the best contribution this person can make?' – both now, through having important work to do, and in the future after appropriate training for making an even more useful contribution.

(4) *Effective use of time*

Good managers know how their time is spent, what is the best use of their time and how to help others use their time well.

(5) *Standards of performance*

Good managers set high standards both for their own work and for the work of others. But for this to be so, a manager must have a clear idea of what such standards are. Standards can range from such things as standards of cleanliness or standards of competence for workers carrying out certain tasks, to standards of coverage of basic health care in the District. Doctors are used to thinking of high standards for clinical work, but the same thinking is needed to determine appropriate standards of managerial and organisational practice throughout the District.

(6) *Clear Objectives*

The way to maintain and improve standards is to set realistic objectives which can be achieved within an identifiable period of time. 'Key result areas' are significant aspects of the District's work to which attention should be given to achieve major improvements in health. Managers also need to relate their personal objectives to those of the organisation as a whole.

(7) *Planning the future whilst managing the present*

Planning is an important management tool, but in practice managers have to plan for the future at the same time as they manage the present. It means not only saying 'What needs to be done now?' but also 'What will need to be done in the future and how should we plan for this now?'. In other words, the good manager uses today's problems and opportunities to create a better future.

(8) *Organising and allocating resources*

The main resources are human, material and financial, as well as time, and the manager's task is to see that these are organised in the most effective way to meet the needs of the District. The manager's skill is in making the fullest use of whatever resources are available. Managers who constantly complain about shortages of money expose their own managerial inefficiency.

(9) *Decision-making*

Bad managers either make bad decisions or none at all. Good managers often make relatively few decisions except those of fundamental importance which have a significant effect on the way in which the District is run. Such decisions establish policies and guidelines within which others can work with the minimum of interference. The manager who is constantly having to make decisions about small matters probably needs to give more thought to policy-making, and to the way work and authority are delegated to others in the District. The timing of decisions is often of the utmost importance. Some decisions are more important than others. In all of them, probably the most critical factor is that of judgement. The wise manager takes advice from other people and sources, and often will look for different points of view, but at the end of the day it is his own judgement of the situation and decisions that matters most.

(10) *Delegating, motivating and developing other people*

One definition of a manager is 'someone who is accountable for more work than he is able to do himself', and who is therefore dependent on other people to do some of that work. This means that a manager must be able to delegate work to others, motivate them and win their commitment, and above all encourage, train and develop others to take on greater responsibilities. The skills the manager needs will include *technical* skills, that is, skills in planning and providing health services; *human* skills, that is, skills of working with people, understanding their problems and getting the best from them; and *balancing* skills, that is, skills of being able to see many factors in a complex situation, assess their relative importance and decide an appropriate course of action.

(11) *Developing and maintaining systems*

Much of the work of a Health District is routine and lends itself to being organised in a systematic way. Such things as the regular supplying of drugs and dressings, the organising of clinic sessions and regular training programmes, need to be based on clear and well-understood systems. A manager needs to review regularly such systems and to adapt them in the light of new circumstances which may arise.

A 'systems approach' uses systems wherever they are appropriate, and to link the various systems together to work smoothly. Care may be needed to develop systems with 'fail-safe' mechanisms, so that work will continue to be done in the most difficult circumstances and if need be by people who have often had minimal education and training.

(12) *Reviewing and evaluating*

Managers will need continually to assess how well the work is being done and what difficulties or problems arise. Much of this can be done on an 'exception' basis, for example identifying exceptionally low or high attendances at clinic or health education sessions. Standards of performance give the manager a very clear idea of the standard of work to be expected. Evaluation and review is far more than the application of certain techniques. It is a whole attitude of mind and style of doing things. Good managers recognise a natural propensity for things to go wrong, as well as often to go right! Any situation therefore is reviewed as a matter of course and corrective action is taken when needed.

(13) *Being an agent of change*

No management situation, especially in the development of Primary Health Care systems, is ever static, and changes are constantly having to be made. Small changes may be made easily in the day to day course of work, but big changes need to be thought out in detail and planned carefully. Management of change is one of the key aspects of a manager's job. Although it is important to maintain a general level of stability in the provision of services within the District, there will be very few times when some significant change or another is not taking place.

Managing within the local socio-cultural environment

To be effective, managers must always work within the limits set by the local environment. In many societies this entails taking into account such things as the social structure of rural life, village decision-making processes, respect for elders, obligations within the extended family, established ways of helping individuals in need, accepted legal and moral codes, and norms of punishment. Together such elements help to make up the way a particular society works and in effect constitute a community's own system of management. An effective health manager therefore needs to work both within this 'local' type of system, and also the type of system with which much of this book is concerned. The manager thus becomes a 'bridge' or an 'integrator' bringing together what is good in both systems to produce a workable means of improving and maintaining the health of the community (see figure 4.9).

Various elements of a District Health Organisation exist in most countries. In some these elements come together to form a viable system with a variable degree of effectiveness. In others the District health system is fragmented with different parts functioning independently and only rarely coming together to influence the health problems. The challenge for the manager of the Health Team is to assemble the various parts of the District Health Organisation into a unified system which can work with efficiency. Some of the principles of creating such a District organisation have been described in this chapter. Only with an adequate District organisation does a mechanism exist for the implementation of the health plans. Without such a mechanism the plans remain only on paper. In the next chapter we go on to discuss how plans can be implemented utilising an effective District health organisation.

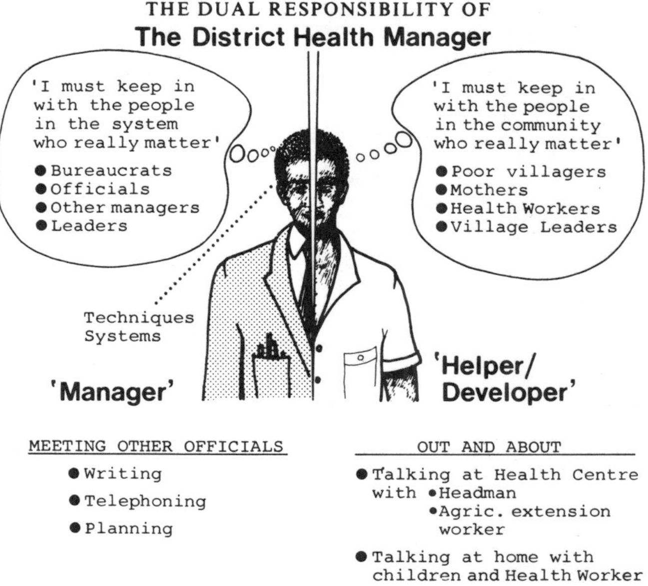

Figure 4.9   The dual responsibility of a district health manager

FURTHER READING

American Public Health Association, *Primary Health Care — progress and problems*, APHA, 1015 15th street, N. W., Washington DC 20005.

Maneno, J., Schluter, P., Sjoerdsma, A. C., Vogel, L. C. and Savage King, F. *Guidelines for the management of hospital outpatient services*, Administrative support Unit, Ministry of Health, Kenya, 1982.

McMahon, R., Barton, E. and Piot, M. *On Being in Charge: A guide for middle-level management in primary health care*, WHO, Geneva, 1980.

5 Practical Management: Putting Plans into Action

Planning should lead to action for achieving results intended in the plan. Managers who have gone through the demanding and difficult exercise of producing a health plan and strategy for their District, develop a strong commitment to putting the plan into practice, but they need all the practical skills and experience available to bring the plan to fruition. However, there are often difficulties. Practical skills are best learnt by doing, and most managers say that they learn how to manage by actually managing. Much of what is called 'management' is common sense and can be recognised as such. This chapter is concerned with what it means to be a manager of a District Health Team concerned with putting a health plan into action. Some techniques will be described which can help managers to organise their own work more efficiently, leading on to a range of issues concerned with managing people, which is at the heart of a manager's work. There is a section concerned with 'logistics' — some of the basic systems which need to work smoothly in a health district; and finally there are practical examples of effective management at three levels — the community, the Health Centre and the District.

MANAGEMENT BY OBJECTIVES

Management by objectives seeks to integrate two things:

(a) the achievement of the aims and purposes of the District Plan (as expressed in the Primary Health Care Plan), with
(b) the need for 'managers' (for example, the District Medical Officer, heads of Health Centres, dispensaries, and so on) to contribute to the aims and objectives of the District Health Plan and to develop skills in their own spheres of work.

It is a demanding and rewarding style of managing a Health District.

When a worthwhile system of 'Management by Objectives' is operating, there is a continuous process of:

(a) critically reviewing and even restating the *long-term and short-term health plans* of the District;

(b) clarifying with each 'manager' his or her *Key Result Areas*, which form part of the District Health Plan;

(c) agreeing with each 'manager' *targets* and *action plans* based on an analysis of the problems and resources available to meet them within each Key Result Area;

(d) providing the right working atmosphere in which managers can achieve their Action Plans; reconciling their objectives with those of others; organising their work; and providing training and support where necessary;

(e) giving *control information* in a form which encourages greater efficiency and better and quicker decision-making;

(f) carrying out *regular reviews* to assess progress made and to develop action plans.

'Management by Objectives' is an important supplement to the *planning* activity in a District since it provides a means of translating plans into action by individual managers. Its use can be illustrated by taking an activity likely to feature in many District Health Plans, for example, that of improving potable water supply. This is likely to be one of the *Key Result Areas* of the manager responsible, say the District Environmental Health and Water Engineer. In practice, managers are not able to deal at any one time with more than a limited number (four or five, and certainly no more than six) Key Result Areas to achieve real results. Key Result Areas emphasise the importance of *results* which are observable, and of measurable improvements within a specified period of time. The Environmental Health and Water Engineer therefore identifies 'improving the supply and use of safe water' as a Key Result Area in his job. Next, he lists the main *problems* in the District which affect the supply and use of safe water to the population, for example,

- seasonal rainfall (six months drought each year);
- water contaminated by refuse, excreta and animals;
- poor wells – uncovered, dirty surrounds, dirty buckets;
- shortage of wells;
- storage containers in villages become contaminated;
- difficulties in transport of water;
- river water also used for drinking, washing, swimming;
- villagers do not understand principles of water hygiene;
- non-availability of pit-privees, and improper use of those available.

He then considers what can be done about each problem, taking into account what resources are available (for example, money, health workers, support and enthusiasm of villagers) and decides on *targets*. The targets need to be *specific* rather than general, and *realistic*, that is, things that in his judgement can be achieved; they should be *measurable* and achievable within a specified *time period*. Thus his targets may include such things as:
Within the next year:

(a) to increase the number of usable wells in the District by 25 per cent;
(b) to make contact with six village development committees and agree with them a programme of maintenance of, for example, wells, walls, covers, hoists and buckets to an acceptable standard;
(c) to bring up to date health education programmes on water use;
(d) to extend the 'water' health education programme to market places and public wells in the District;
(e) to contact riverside villages and agree programmes for better use of available water;
(f) to finalise above plans with Public Works Department and prepare budget estimates;
(g) to increase the number of sanitarians in the District from 20 to 25;
(h) to provide basic training for newly-appointed sanitarians and refresher training for all others.

With the help of such targets the Water Engineer has a very clear idea of what is to be achieved during the next year, and can organise his work accordingly. This can be done by listing against each of the targets the precise action to be taken, and who will take it. In this way he produces objectives for each of his staff. In the course of the year the Water Engineer will need to check regularly to see what progress is being made to achieve these targets and will need to visit widely within the District to receive *control information* in the form of regular reports from sanitarians, Health Centres, and so on. This feedback of information is important as it enables objectives to be revised where necessary and updated for succeeding years.

Table 5.1 shows a way of setting out the kind of information needed for this type of approach, using the example of the Environmental Health and Water Engineer just discussed.

To be successful a manager should agree objectives in conjunction with other people. Thus in the above example, the District Water Engineer would agree his broad objectives and targets with other members of the District Health Team, thereby benefiting from their ideas, as well as ensuring that his objectives are compatible with theirs. Such an exercise also helps to strengthen the commitment of all concerned. Similarly, by discussing and agreeing targets with the sanitarians, health workers, and others who work for him, he can explain why certain work has to be done, how it contributes to the

Table 5.1   Example of method of setting out kind of information needed for Environmental Health and Water Engineer in district

NAME: JOB TITLE: LOCATION: DATE:

.... Environmental Health Officer   .... Health District   March 1983

Key result area	Problems	Resources available to meet problems	Targets	Action plans	Means of control/review
Improve the supply and use of safe water	*Water sources* . Seasonal rainfall . Poor wells . Shortage of wells	1. *Finance* Annual budget +10% special allocation	. Increase number of useable wells by 25%	. Agree location . Allocate layout . Supervise progress	Monthly return on number of wells in use
	Distribution and supply . Poor storage . Transport difficulties	2. *Staff* Environmental Health Workers Other Health Workers	. Start programme with six village health committees	. Discuss with District Medical Officer . Draw up outline programme . Arrange meetings	Reports from village health committees
	Human Waste Disposal . Mixed use of rivers . Ignorance of water hygiene . Shortage of latrines . Contaminated wells	3. *Other support* Villagers Schools Market Superintendents 4. Public Works Department	. Update Health Education Programme	. Discuss with Provincial Water Engineer . Get help of Training School	Completed programme by. . . ..
			. Extend Health Education Programme to markets and wells	. Contact market superintendents and headmen . Train health educators	Reports from market superintendents Inspection of wells

. Agree programme with riverside villages	. Inspect rivers . Report to headmen . Agree programme	Reports from riverside headmen
Finalise plans with . Public Works Dept. for drilling wells	. Agree programme and budget with Public Works Department . Monitor progress	Monthly reports from Public Works Department
. Increase number of sanitarians by 25%	. Agree establishment and budget . Recruit from schools and villages	Numbers in post
. Provide basic and refresher training	. Update training programme . Allocate trainers . Fix training dates	Numbers of trained 'graduates'

improvement of health, and thus provide an opportunity for his staff to contribute ideas and share in the planning and running of environmental health work in the District.

As a technique, management by objectives becomes really effective where it is linked to other systems in the District. It is a natural way of translating ideas from the *planning* system into the action system; where objectives are carefully costed it becomes part of the *financial control* system; it is a basis for the District's *Work Allocation* system; it provides a base for realistic policies for *recruitment, training and development* of staff in the District. In some organisations its use has been taken to extremes, but used sensibly it is a technique which can help managers to tackle the day to day work and the future development of the District in a systematic way.

STANDARDS

The question of standards is central to any consideration of Management by Objectives and indeed to the work of a manager. Whether consciously or not, managers are continually making judgements about standards in their day to day work. Such statements as 'X' has done a good job, 'Supplies have been arriving late during the past month', 'Too few patients are attending this clinic', 'We are making good progress in digging new wells', each refer to a standard of some kind. There is a standard of work which is expected of 'X'; a standard of punctuality expected for receiving supplies; some idea (or standard) of the number of patients who ought to attend a clinic; some measure or target for digging new wells in the locality. Managers who set high standards for themselves and constantly work to improve those standards, are in the best position to require and obtain high standards of work from others, provided that those standards are realistic. What is more important is for managers to set realistic standards agreed and accepted by those whose duty it is to implement them. Standards should as far as possible be measurable with regard to:

Quantity	(for example, the number of patients to be seen in a clinic session)
Quality	(for example, the quality of care provided and hence the need for written procedures for routine treatment and emergencies)
Cost	(for example, average drug cost per patient for common illnesses)
Time	(for example, time taken per patient consultation)

Such standards need to be taken into account in assessing how well a health facility is run. Other standards for a health facility might include:

Access	for example, 80 per cent of the local population have access to services; 75 per cent of expectant mothers receive antenatal care (next year we aim to raise this to 85 per cent) No patient has to wait more than one hour to be seen, and 70 per cent are seen within 30 minutes.
History-taking	A history is taken of every patient, which answers at least three of the questions in the Medical Assistant's Manual.
Examination	Every patient is examined before a diagnosis is made.

The following are Effectiveness Standards for Primary Health Care which may be adopted by a District Health Team:

(1) Nothing is done at a higher level of health provision (for example, District hospital) which can be done equally well at a lower level (for example, health centre or village).
(2) Until such time as basic health care needs are met a significant proportion (say 50 per cent) of the District's total budget will be spent at Levels A and B.
(3) A significant proportion of time (20–50 per cent) of those with skills at Levels B and C will be spent in training others.
(4) Services provided at Level A, and a proportion (up to 30 per cent) at Level B, will be provided in response to and with the support of villagers, usually expressed through a Village Health Committee.
(5) No major item of spending or change of plan will be incurred by one function (Medical, Nursing, Environmental Health) without the positive agreement of all the District Health Team.

Obviously these are only examples of standards which might be acceptable, and there are limits to having detailed standards for every conceivable situation. What is needed is for health workers and managers to have a clear idea of the standard of work expected. Standards of work are often low because it has never been made clear what level of performance is expected.

In summary, where managers think through in a systematic way as to what objectives and targets they can achieve in future, they are more likely to achieve them; and where standards of performance and work are made clear to workers involved, there is a greater likelihood of improved standards being achieved.

PERSONAL SKILLS OF THE MANAGER

Managing time

As managers, members of the District Health Team are concerned with the effective management of the health programme of the District as a whole. But management must start with the effective personal management of each member of the team. Their own time and the use they make of it is one of the single most important assets to the District.

Generally speaking, Health Managers have learnt by experience during their professional training how to plan and use time in order to study and fulfil clinical commitments as well as maintain social and family life. Now, as managers, a new aspect of managing time becomes important. There can be a constant conflict between professional and managerial roles. By inclination and training physicians may be equipped to treat and care for individuals, yet the job requires them to have a concern for the health of communities and increasingly to manage the work of others rather than do clinical work themselves. A first step to resolving the conflict is to analyse how time is actually spent. This can be done on both a long-term and a short-term basis.

On a long-term basis, consider how you have spent your time during, say, the previous 12 months, and quantify in percentage terms, as accurately as possible, how much time has been spent on, for example:

- Clinical work with individual patients
- Work in hospital, health centres and dispensaries
- Time spent in planning and assessing health needs in the community
- Time spent with other health workers, helping them to do their work better
- Travelling
- Management and administrative tasks
- Study and keeping up to date professionally
- Personal and free time

Then think carefully about the nature of your job priorities in the Health District, the most effective contribution you can make, and priorities for your own work. This should result in a changed set of percentage time for most of the elements into which you have broken down your work. Many doctors who have done this exercise have found that they need to give more attention to the development and managerial aspects of their work than to clinical and routine administrative work. The problem is how to do it and where to find the time!

There are a number of ways of coping with the problem:

(a) Learn to say 'no'. Many of the demands on time are made by other people, and ways can be found to say 'no' or to minimise those demands if they do not contribute to the achievement of your own priorities. Unfortunately it is often easier to respond to other people's demands than to establish one's own priorities and work on those. Of course, some demands are important and people must not be sent away without due consideration. Here a simple motto to follow is: 'Be gracious with people, but ruthless with time'.

(b) Delegate. Effective managers ask of every piece of work that comes to them 'who else could do this?'. They do not work themselves out of a job in this way, but create time to concentrate on the more important aspects of their work, and also create opportunities for others to take on more responsibility.

(c) Make arrangements with colleagues for rational distribution of work. If the problem is that too much time is being spent in doing clinical work in the main hospital in the District, then it may mean starting discussions with other doctors in the hospital or with the hospital authorities about the importance of rural health programmes in relation to hospital work, and agreeing new patterns of work.

(d) Plan specific 'periods' of time to do specific jobs – for example, for the first half-hour of every Monday plan the week's work with colleagues, and for the first three weeks in the month spend every Friday afternoon developing the training strategy for the District.

(e) Develop a heightened awareness of time through use of a systematic 'Diary Review', such as that shown in Figure 5.1. Note down systematically over a two-week period, every half-hour during the working day, precisely what you are doing, and then analyse the results. You will probably be surprised by how you have actually spent your time compared with how you think you have spent it. A change in daily and weekly allocations of time should follow.

(f) Have monthly, weekly and daily lists of priorities. Many managers write down each morning a 'Things to do' list and keep it on their desk or in their pocket marking items as A, B or C priorities. By working on priority A items as far as possible despite the inevitable interruptions, they usually end each day having achieved most, if not all, of the important things they had hoped to do.

(g) Have the question 'How could I *now* be best using my time?' frequently in mind. This can prevent time being spent on unimportant matters at the expense of more productive concerns.

(h) Help other workers in the District to examine critically the use of their time, so that they pay maximum attention to the most important aspects of the health programme. Time studies at clinics may identify much more effective ways for clinics to be organised and health workers to spend their time. Time studies in themselves can also be a means of evaluating health centre work.

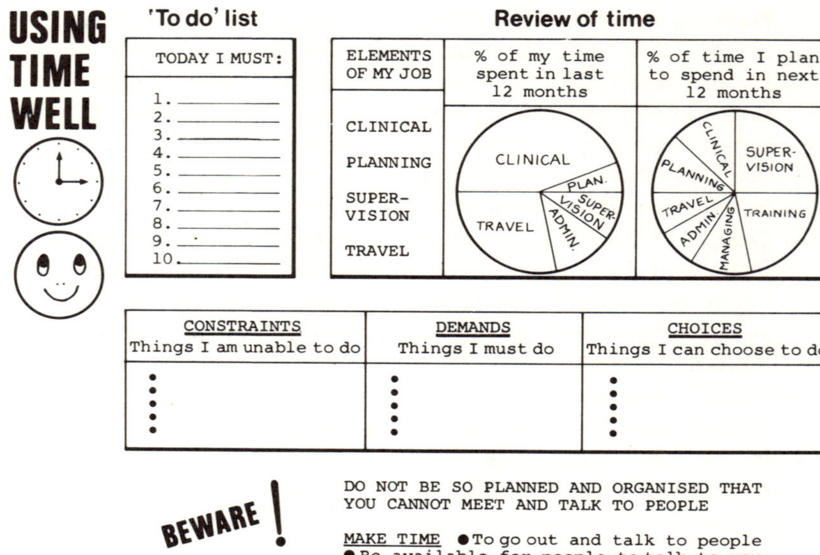

Figure 5.1   Using time well

(i) Examine travelling time. Unnecessary travel not only wastes time but also keeps vehicles on the road more often than is necessary resulting in excessive use of fuel and more wear and tear. If travel is co-ordinated, two or more people can travel in one vehicle if they have assignments to perform at the same place or on the same route. Moreover, members of staff of the same health facility can have consultations and discuss problems among themselves during group travel.

(j) Think carefully about meetings. The larger the meeting, the more time is being spent at it, therefore make sure that all meetings serve a useful purpose. Have an agenda circulated well ahead in time and for important matters ask for discussion papers to be prepared. Develop also the skills needed for effective meetings so that time is not wasted on minor issues and serious matter is not neglected for lack of time.

(k) Analyse your time into Demands (things I must do), Constraints (things I am not able to do) and Choices (things I can choose to do). Consider what a wide range of choices may be open to you, before finally deciding how to spend your time.

A final word of caution, however, is needed. A rural community can have its own pace of life which is very different from that of a brisk and bustling urban community. An effective Rural Health Team needs to gear its activities to the pace of the community it serves, and much time may need to be spent in a community to build trust and understanding. Such time should be planned for and given a high priority.

Delegation

Reference has been made to this important aspect of a manager's work in chapter 3. It is proposed to discuss delegation in greater detail now.

A District Medical Officer or manager of the health team responsible for all the work of a District must of necessity delegate a great deal of work to others in the organisation. The skills of effective delegation are high-order skills for senior managers, and need to be practised continually if the Health District as an organisation is to run smoothly.

The advantages of delegation are that it gives to those who delegate more time to do the things which only they can do. It makes fuller use of people's skills and abilities which would otherwise be wasted. It enables subordinates to identify themselves more closely with the aims of the organisation, and thus to feel more responsible. It increases the total capacity of the organisation without increasing resources. It gives staff generally more job satisfaction and opportunity to learn, and it ensures that there are capable people able to act in the manager's absence (see figure 5.2).

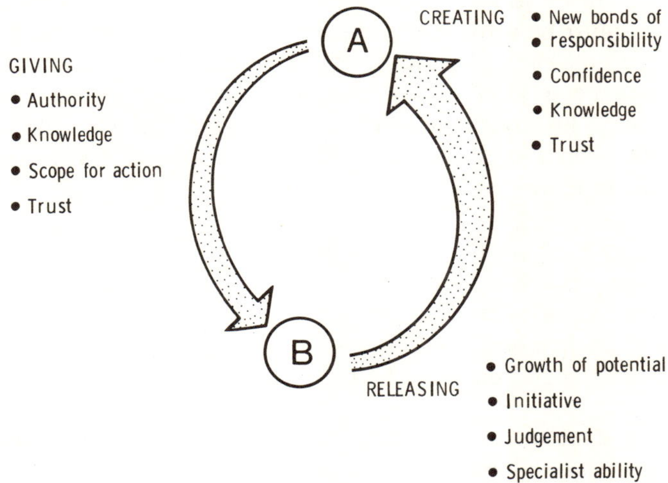

Figure 5.2   What happens when A delegates successfully to B

There are risks in delegation as in everything else, and these deter senior staff from delegating more work and authority to their subordinates. A senior manager is still accountable for the proper performance of those tasks which have been delegated to a subordinate. For example, a District Medical Officer may in practice delegate the day-to-day running of a Health Centre or a dispensary to a Primary Health Worker who is on the spot, but is still accountable to his superiors for the services provided in the Centre. A golden rule is that a manager can delegate work and authority to carry out work, but he can never delegate his own responsibility and accountability for that work — the buck stops with the senior manager. The manager then is still responsible for mistakes made by a subordinate, yet may feel loss of control over the work, at the same time being ignorant of much of the details of the work of which he was previously knowledgeable. There may also be a deeper fear that the subordinate will become more competent at certain aspects of the work — there is evidence for example that medical assistants can be more efficient at diagnosing certain common conditions by the use of algorithms or flow charts than doctors using more established and conventional methods of diagnosis. Again, the senior manager may feel under pressure from other staff to delegate to them more responsibility before they are ready for it.

Certain conditions need to exist for effective delegation to occur. There needs to be a relationship of trust between the persons concerned. The person delegating must feel sure that the person to whom work is being delegated is competent; the person being delegated to must feel free to ask for help when it is needed. The work being delegated and what is to be achieved by it must be clearly defined to the satisfaction of both parties, and the subordinate given full authority to do it. Any training necessary for the performance of new assignments must be provided, and such supervision as may be necessary, particularly in the early stages of the work, should be forthcoming. But the most important condition is for the subordinate to feel free to get on with the work without feeling over-controlled or constrained, and to receive full credit for the work when it has been done well. The subordinate really asks for five things of his superiors:

1. Agree with me clearly what I should do.
2. Give me a real chance to do it.
3. Give me knowledge of my progress.
4. Give me help when I need it.
5. Give me recognition when I have done it.

Controls and methods of reporting back should be agreed. This can be done by agreeing what standards of work apply, and agreeing how the work is to be checked against those standards. Then when variations in standard occur, the causes of the variation can be identified and corrective action taken to remedy the situation. An example would be where a health worker in charge of a rural dispensary is delegated authority to dispense a certain drug up to a limit of, say, 1000 mg a week. Were he to prescribe more than that amount in any one week, the variation would be sanctioned by a more senior health worker, and the reasons investigated. It could be that the health worker is dispensing too much for each patient, or for the wrong condition, or that there is a genuine increase in need for that treatment. Whatever the reason, action can be taken either to give more instruction or training to the health worker or, if necessary, to alter the standard of 1000 mg. Such a system of delegation and control can be a powerful deterrant to malpractices such as misuse or selling of drugs. It gives the health workers freedom to work within limits which are reasonable so far as their training and experience are concerned.

TEAMWORK

In chapter 4 a District organisation was looked at as a skill pyramid, as a series of interrelated groups, and as a network of relationships. The success of the health activities in the District depends to a large extent on people working well together in small groups, and those small groups relating well to one another.

In an established District there can be anywhere between 40 and 100 working teams (see table 5.2) and senior management will have a direct involvement or interest in nearly all of them. Where the organisational structure is hierarchical it becomes critically important to try and organise horizontal relationships between the different agencies, through a process of team work. Orientation is needed for various staff to help them co-ordinate their efforts to bring about an improvement in the health status of the community as a whole. Definition of tasks is helpful for plotting out exactly where activities need to be co-ordinated. Training sessions are needed to help existing health providers acquire the skills necessary for performing specified tasks, the aim being to produce practical multi-purpose health providers rather than uni-purpose ones, trained as much together as possible and within the environment in which they are going to work. Managers who take on this task of team-building will recognise the following features of effective working teams:

(1) A clear *purpose* and *common task* which everyone in the group understands and is committed to. Managers need to help each group to appreciate what its own function is and how it fits into the over-all work of the District.
(2) Each member of the group has *a clear idea of his or her own job* and how it relates to the work of others.
(3) Individual members of the group *understand the work and duties of others*, particularly where there is overlap in functions (for example, a nurse and medical assistant may each do similar work from time to time). Where members must be able to replace one another or overlap in their functions, this understanding is strengthened by having multi-purpose workers, particularly at village and health centre levels.
(4) *Flexibility* between members is helpful so that the work of the team does not collapse when one member is absent.

Table 5.2 **Pattern of organisation in an established district**

Description	Number	Approximate no. in working group	Membership of working group	Function/purpose
Rural Dispensaries	20–80	3–6	Rural dispensary assistant Village health worker (male) Village health worker (female) (Traditional birth attendants (2)) Cleaner Nurse aide	First level of Health Care: . Community development . Diagnosis . Treatment . Referral to Health Centre . Health education . Immunisations . Sanitation
Health Centres	2–4	8–11	Medical assistant/Doctor Rural medical aid Village midwife 2 Community nurses Lab. technician Sanitarian Registration clerk 3 Cleaners/Aux. Staff	Second level of Health Care
District Mobile Team	1	5–6	District Medical Officer Nurse/Midwife 2 Medical recorders 1 Nurse student Driver	Supervision of Health Centres Clinics Health education

District Management Team	1	3–4	District Medical Officer Matron Hospital Administrator Hospital Finance Officer	Management of all District Health Services Executive of Health Authority
Hospital Management Board	1	12+		
Hospital Doctors	1	3–4	District Medical Officer 1–2 Physicians 1–2 Surgeons	Diagnosis & treatment Training & support to all health workers
Hospital Wards & Departments	10	6–8	Ward sister Physician or Surgeon Nurses Auxiliaries Attendants/Cleaners	Care & treatment of patients

(5) This suggests that a good deal of *learning* and *training will go on* within the team, encouraged and stimulated by the team leader.

(6) *Leadership*. In most working teams the leader is clearly identifiable as the person in charge. In some teams (for example, a working group set up to achieve a specific task) the leader may not be formally appointed, but someone will need to take on the leadership function, even if the leadership role changes depending on the task in hand. For instance, a doctor may normally be the leader of an outreach team but when the same team goes out to run antenatal clinics it may be a midwife or community nurse who takes charge. Good leaders are recognised as such by the rest of the team.

(7) *Stability and continuity*. If the members of a group continue changing there can hardly ever be teamwork. On the other hand, a group which never changes its membership may become set in its ways and complacent.

(8) An effective group needs sufficient *resources* to carry out its task (these need not be costly as is the case with much of Primary Health Care) and it needs its own *working methods* and *procedures* which are well understood and practised.

(9) Good *relationships* within the group are vital and require openness, understanding and a willingness to help. Amongst the team manager's most important skills are those of human relations – the art of building and strengthening good relationships with and between others.

(10) The real test of a team's success is its results, so it is important to have ways of measuring success and recognising achievement.

(11) *Loyalty*. An effective team develops a strong sense of cohesion and loyalty which enables it to work well and often to tackle new problems successfully. But this loyalty should not be at the expense of other groups. Groups need to co-operate with others, and frequently people will be members of more than one group (for example, a nurse who works in both a Health Centre and with other nurses in the district). The District Medical Officer has a key part to play in overcoming the dangers of groups working in isolation by explaining and interpreting the functions of particular parts of the health organisation to other parts, and seeing that the work of the total organisation is well balanced and understood.

This can be done through 'linking-pins' in the organisation. Groups working at different levels in a District can be linked together through the involvement of one member in each group in the work of another group at a different level in the organisation. Thus, each Rural Dispensary Aide (RDA) is a leader of health workers at the village level, and may also be made a member of a team at the Health Centre, headed by a Medical Assistant, which includes other Rural Dispensary Aides and key Health Centre staff. The Rural Dispensary

Aides thus provide a vital link between the two levels of health care —
to ensure that Health Centre staff understand the needs of those
working at the village level, and that members of the village teams
understand how the Health Centre works and deals with patients
referred from the village. The Rural Dispensary Aides should also
from time to time meet with 'colleagues' working in other villages to
share ideas on how they run their dispensaries. Similarly, Rural
Medical Assistants act as a link between Health Centre and District
levels of care.

Meetings

Regular staff meetings are amongst the important tools of management and
may be held to discuss common problems, review progress, plan future work,
and so on. Handled well, they can produce great benefits, but run badly,
meetings can lead to frustration, acrimony and poor results.

Many meetings flounder because little thought goes into them either
beforehand or during the meeting itself. There are some simple tips, however,
which can help run a meeting successfully. These can be summarised as the 5
'p's:

> Planning
> Pre-notification
> Preparation
> Processing
> Putting it on record

Planning

Think through the purpose of the meeting in advance, and what it is intended
to achieve.

Pre-notification

Inform other members of the meeting what is to be discussed and why, so that
they can come properly prepared.

Preparation

Arrange an agenda in its proper sequence and allot the correct amount of time
for each subject. Give more time to the more important issues.

Processing

Structure the discussion of each item, to keep members on the point, and to
avoid the pitfalls of repeatedly covering old ground; develop a consciousness

of group behaviour, control private discussions, and reconcile disagreements within the group.

Putting it on record

Summarise and record decisions made and action to be taken.

Group effectiveness assessment

A 'Group Effectiveness Assessment' is a simple chart which can be used by a team leader, or members of a working group, to gain insight into the workings of a group. All the members of a group are asked to give their views on each of the nine variables and one can see where the low and the high ratings occur. Low ratings may indicate the need for change; high ratings may indicate features to be built on and strengthened.

Group effectiveness assessment

Analyse your group by rating it on a scale from 1 to 7 (7 being what you consider to be the ideal) with respect to each of these variables:

(1) *Group Objectives*
   (a) Not understood by group — (1)———(7) Clearly understood by group
   (b) Group is negative towards objectives — (1)———(7) Group is committed to objectives

(2) *Utilisation of member resources*
   Our abilities, knowledge and experience aren't fully utilised as a group — (1)———(7) Our abilities, knowledge and experience are fully utilised

(3) *Degree of mutual support*
   High suspicion — (1)———(7) High trust

(4) *Control methods*
   Control is imposed on us — (1)———(7) We control ourselves

(5) *Handling conflicts within group*
   We deny, avoid or suppress conflicts — (1)———(7) We accept conflicts and work them through

(6) *Experimental Learning*
   We ignore and do not learn from our group experiences — ———(7) We analyse our experience and learn about group growth

(7) *Organisational environment*
   Restrictive; pressure for   (1)————(7)   Free, supportive,
   conformity   respect for differences

(8) *Communications*
   (a) Guarded, cautious   (1)————(7)   Open, authentic
   (b) We don't listen to   (1)————(7)   We listen, we understand
       each other   and are understood

(9) *Sense of belonging*
   No cohesiveness. We have (1)————(7)   We have a sense of
   no sense of belonging   belonging to the group.
                                                          We want to work in it.

MOTIVATION

One of the most important resources available to the Health District is the working potential of those employed within it. But it is often said that those involved in rural health care are under-employed, disinterested in their work, and not prepared to put into their work more than the minimum that is required.

The motivation of physicians working in rural areas is important since the attitudes of those in positions of leadership have a considerable influence on the attitudes of others. When students in a number of medical schools in India were interviewed it was found that amongst their positive attitudes were: the opportunities rural health work would give them to provide medical care to communities, to give services to needy people, to offer preventive and curative services as a package of comprehensive care, to have independent responsibility and to meet national needs. What they disliked about work in rural areas was the lack of educational opportunities for their children, the lack of adequate supplies of drugs and equipment, the lack of opportunity for their own professional development (for example, lack of postgraduate education, libraries, and so on), the isolation and lack of transport to urban areas, and lastly, the relatively poor pay and conditions of service.

Similar studies could be made of other health workers, but even without such detailed studies a District Medical Officer or management team should be aware of the attitudes and motivation of workers within the district. Lists can be drawn up of factors about which rural health workers have positive attitudes (motivators) and a list of the factors about which they feel badly (de-motivators). Such a list is shown in table 5.3.

Table 5.3 only shows examples of what *may* be found as attitudes amongst health workers in rural areas. They may vary considerably from place to place. Implications for a District Health Manager are clear – if the negative aspects of the job remain, the morale and enthusiasm of the health workers and of

Table 5.3 **Attitudes of health workers in rural areas**

Motivators (positive aspects of the job)	*De-motivators (negative aspects of the job)*
Opportunity to improve the health of the local community.	Isolation, especially when not quite sure what to do.
Status – being held in high regard by the local community.	Having to work without proper supplies (drugs, equipment, etc.).
Future prospects – the opportunity to learn more and gain better paid and more responsible work in the future.	Fear of making mistakes which could affect patients' lives.
Independence and responsibility.	Boredom and routine.
Working in a team with other people.	Conflicting pressures (e.g. by DMO to limit over-prescribing, and from villagers to provide drugs which are not really needed).
Financial security of a regular paid job. The security of doing routine work with clearly laid down procedures.	

those with whom they come into contact will deteriorate. Action must be taken to remedy the negative aspects (for example, better arrangements for drug supplies, refresher courses, better professional support, and so on). At the same time the positive aspects of the job need to be reinforced, as these are the aspects which encourage the health workers to work with enthusiasm and put as much as they can into their work.

In considering motivation it is helpful to look at the more fundamental reasons why people work. Two sets of attitudes to work, 'Theory X' and 'Theory Y', have been described as follows and illustrated in table 5.4.

Theory X
(1) The average human being has an inherent dislike of work and will avoid it if he can.
(2) Because of this human characteristic of dislike of work, most people must be coerced, controlled, directed, or threatened with punishment to get them to put forth adequate effort towards the achievement of organisational objectives.
(3) The average human being prefers to be directed, wishes to avoid responsibility, has relatively little ambition, and wants security above all.

Theory Y
(1) Work is as natural as play or rest. Depending upon *controllable conditions*, it may be a source of satisfaction (and will be voluntarily performed) or a source of revulsion (and will be avoided if possible).
(2) External control and punishment are not the only means of achieving

effort. Man will exercise self-direction and self-control in the services of objectives to which he is committed.

(3) Personal satisfaction can be the direct product of effort directed towards organisational objectives.

(4) Most people, under proper conditions, learn not only to accept but to seek responsibility. Avoidance of responsibility, lack of ambition, and emphasis *on security are generally consequences of experience and lack of it but not inherent human characteristics.*

(5) The capacity to exercise creativity in solving problems is widely distributed in the population. But under modern working conditions, the intellectual potential of the average human being is only partially utilised.

'Theory X' attitudes are quite prevalent, and particularly relate to those who have to carry out more menial tasks. How can the conditions of 'Theory Y' apply to, say, a sweeper who is employed to keep the floors and surrounding of a Health Centre or dispensary clean, hygienic and tidy? Yet there are many examples of people who have been encouraged to do this kind of work well, through praise, being helped to feel part of the Health Centre team, and having a clear idea of the standard of work required. Such people have responded by extending the limits of their work, taking on new tasks and finding new ways to be helpful. Similarly well-motivated and effective working teams often look for ways of improving their own work and look for new and challenging tasks to achieve.

District Health Managers therefore need to think carefully about their own motivation. They must have a genuine desire to improve the health of the district population; they must believe that the job is worth doing, and can be achieved; have faith in their own abilities to achieve it; and have clear goals and strategies to bring it about. They must also be able to motivate other people to share in the task. This may be done in different ways with different people – with professional colleagues it may be by working with them, persuading and 'selling' ideas in meetings, seminars and committees; with other health workers by good organisation, supporting and encouraging them; with village workers and leaders in the community by understanding, listening, co-operating and helping; and with the mass of ordinary people in the community by helping, educating and encouraging them to cope with their own lives and health problems.

COMMUNICATION

Good communication is the corner stone of any strategy of rural health care. Village health workers identify major health needs by observing, listening and

Table 5.4 **Two sets of attitudes to work**

Theory X *Manager*	*Theory Y* *Manager*
'I am not really interested in this job – My workers are lazy and idle; they only work if I threaten to discipline or "bribe" them; they do not want to better themselves; they avoid responsibility; they don't want to do anything new.'	'We have a difficult job to do here but we are making some progress – My workers enjoy their work: I explain clearly what I want them to do, give them whatever help they need and praise them when they do it well; I trust them to work well on their own because I know they will do it; they get a lot of satisfaction from doing their work well – I encourage them to take more responsibility and they do so; they frequently solve their own problems and often help me solve my own; I do whatever I can to help them achieve their own goals.'
Result: Workers sitting around, sulky, no initiative, work not done properly. Health Centre dirty and badly organised. Workers afraid of the manager and keep out of the way.	*Result*: Workers very active. Well run Health Centre. Many village activities. Workers, managers and villagers work together on new projects. Workers have new ideas and put them into practice.

talking with villagers; the relationship between patient and health worker is one of dialogue, with both parties listening and trying to understand what the other is saying; qualified staff in supervising others do not just tell them what to do, but adopt a problem-solving approach, discussing problems together and jointly agreeing solutions.

Much of medical and health worker training has been based on the assumption that those who have health knowledge are 'experts' and must pass on their 'expertise' to others. This of course is only half the story. The village health workers are the experts on their own village, knowing the history and village traditions, the personalities of the villagers and relationships between them; the particular problems such as water shortage, crop disease, and infections that villagers have to face. Workers in the Health Centre are the experts on the Health Centre and its problems, the needs of the population it serves. Health Managers need to take in this information as well as to give out their own expertise. So they need to be experts at listening as well as at passing on their expertise. This is communication. It often means working with whatever channels of communication are available.

It is useful to map out the Communication System of a District along the lines shown in table 5.5 and see how it links with information and other systems. By thinking carefully about formal communication flow, gaps and duplications may be eliminated. At the same time informal communications must never be forgotten. However much formal communication systems are improved, managers need to be aware of the vast amount of information which is communicated informally and should remain close enough to people to 'pick up' what is being said and felt around the District.

Managers find that up to 90 per cent of their working time can be spent in communicating. The essential elements of communication are listening, talking, reading and writing. Yet for most of the time they are hardly aware that they are communicating. Much of their work is accomplished by talking with individuals. Increasingly, managers need to discuss with groups of people, which entails careful listening if all the things that people may be trying to say are to be understood, and of course careful speaking if the manager is to get his own point of view over successfully. The larger the group, the more 'public speaking' skills are needed, besides those of encouraging others, reconciling different points of view and explaining complex issues. Writing skills are important, particularly in dealing with higher levels of government and other organisations. Where literacy levels are low, care must be given to simple, clear and unambiguous writing. A great deal of communication, however, takes place at a level beyond the spoken or written word, and is concerned more with feelings and emotions. It is expressed in looks, bodily gestures, silences. Skilled listeners take these factors into account at the same time as hearing the actual words which are used.

Table 5.5 **Example of part of a Communications Chart for a District**

Communicator	Method	How often	Items for discussion	Purpose	Length
District Medical Officer or District Management Team	Meeting and Action Sheet	Weekly/ Fortnightly	District Strategy, District Resources, Activities/Evaluation Common Problems Priorities	To ensure a concerted approach to management of the District	1–2 hrs
District Medical Officer and Health Centre Supervisor	Meeting individually and with Health Centre staff	Monthly	Previous month's work Unusual referrals to District Hospital Problems Priorities for next month	Supervision and support of Health Centre Supervisor. Link with Health Centre	2–3 hrs
Health Centre Supervisor and staff	Meeting	Weekly	Priorities Problems Allocation of work Matters to discuss with District Medical Officer	To ensure a team approach in the Health Centre	20/30 min
Health Centre Supervisor and village health workers	Meeting or individually in village	Monthly	Problems in the village Training and supervision referrals	To support village health workers and ensure Health Centre meets the needs of villagers	2–3 hrs
Health Centre Supervisor, village health worker and village development committee (& District Medical Officer for major problems or issues)	Meeting	3-monthly	Previous 3 month's work Problems Links between Health and other projects	To ensure continued support and commitment of Village Development Committee	1–2 hrs

MANAGEMENT OF CHANGE

From time to time situations arise in a Health District which indicate the need for change. The whole process of implementing a health plan requires change. The long-term aim of the health plan may be to get the people to change their daily living habits with regard to feeding, hygiene, child-care or self-care. As new health needs in the community are identified, health workers will need to change their ways of working in order to meet them. Profound changes may be needed in the balance between hospital and Primary Health Care. Within the primary health sector, change may be essential because of staff changes. Fresh ideas and new knowledge may require changes in strategy. The District Health Team frequently has the job of bringing about and implementing change in the District. Individual managers achieve changes in different ways, but always a balance has to be struck between trying to change too much or too little, trying to change too quickly or too slowly, and bringing about changes with the support and consent of the people as well as of the workers involved. Leadership must suggest and demonstrate new ways of doing things, but a good leader does not get so far ahead of people that changes and new approaches are misunderstood and resented. Managers can have the greatest problems where there is resistance to change.

People usually react to change from the standpoint of 'What's in it for me?' and it is therefore important to see changes from the point of view of those who will be affected.

Where people are resistant to change, they may show it through being less interested in work, sometimes 'opting out' of their responsibilities, sometimes refusing to accept that the change will take place, or complaining more about their work. In some cases people become much more dependent or antagonistic to supervisors or those they think are trying to bring about the changes. They may continue to do things in the same way as before, particularly if it is a long-established practice or if they have been well trained to work that way. In addition, if a number of individuals feel threatened by change, they are likely to strengthen themselves as a group to resist the change.

Many of these reactions will be found familiar. Take the case of a Health Centre which has been established for a number of years but which has failed to adapt during that period to changes in population, income and expectation of services amongst the population it serves. The result is that many people no longer come to the Health Centre – expectant mothers and 'at risk' groups do not attend preventive and education programmes; those with minor ailments bypass the Health Centre and go to a more distant rural hospital for treatment; Health Centre staff dispense larger and larger amounts of drugs for cases which do not really need them, mainly to show that they are busy. Along comes a bright new medical officer who decides that changes are needed. Imagine the feelings and reactions of the Health Centre Supervisor whose reactions may be defensive: 'Why change? – we have always done it this way'; he may withdraw support by refusing to meet or communicate openly with the new medical officer; he may even be critical or apathetic to whatever new ideas are put forward. One can also see how such resistance would spread to other workers at the centre and to members of the community as well.

How might the medical officer respond to such resistance? An immediate response, but one not likely to succeed, might be:

Defence – reacting to the resistance as a personal attack and asserting his authority as the medical officer,
Persuasion – attempting simply to argue with the supervisor without recognising what feelings are involved.
Criticising the way the Health Centre has been run in the past.
Control – seeking to force change on the Health Centre.
Punishment – threatening punishment or withholding rewards if the changes are not made.

A more successful approach would be to:

Attempt to understand the feelings of the superintendent and other workers and avoid inappropriate actions.
Create an atmosphere of confidence and trust that will minimise resistance, increase understanding and secure co-operation.
Communicate. Encourage the staff to talk about their problems and discuss what actions may help to solve them. Explain why change is needed.
Gain the confidence of those affected by the change through involvement and participation. The more the staff are involved in planning change, the less they will resist it.
Get the right timing. Slow changes can be easier than rapid ones, since this gives people time to adjust, but it can also be unsettling if the change is too long drawn out.
Reassure staff that training and support will be available to enable them to cope with any new situations which may arise.
Be flexible. Be prepared to accept modifications if these are seen to be desirable. There are usually a number of ways to achieve the same ends.
Succeed! All successful handling of change engenders confidence and trust. The next change to be made will be that much easier.

INTRODUCING CHANGE

There is no one systematic approach for introducing change. Organisations and managers are different and there are many different factors to take into account. This checklist may, however, serve as a useful guide to managing change.

Recognising the need for change

(1) What is the objective of the change?
(2) What data do I have to support the need for change?
(3) Do others need to be convinced of the need for change? How can I achieve this?
(4) Am I sure that the need for change will not be met by other developments?

Planning the change

(1) What is the best method for accomplishing the change? Can other methods be used, provided that the objectives are achieved?
(2) Should a pilot change programme be tried first?
(3) Is the present organisation sufficiently flexible to accept change?
(4) Is there a deadline for achieving the change? Is this deadline flexible?
(5) Do I have the involvement and commitment of people who matter, for example, community leaders, senior officials?
(6) Can I introduce the change myself or should some other individual or group be used as the change agent?
(7) What will be the effects of change on other parts of the organisation?
(8) Have I considered the reaction of individuals which may act as a barrier to the change?
(9) Is the change programme clear?

Implementing the change

(1) Is the responsibility for the change programme being placed at a sufficiently senior level?
(2) How can I obtain commitment from others to the new objectives?
(3) How can I maintain momentum in the change programme?
(4) Are those responsible for introducing the change acceptable to others?
(5) Will the change, once achieved, meet expectations aroused in the organisation?
(6) If time and energy are to be devoted to achieving the change, have I made arrangement so that my normal work activities are not neglected during the period of implementing the change?
(7) What are the means to be used to ensure that the new way of doing things is maintained?

Checking and monitoring change

(1) What quantitative and qualitative data am I collecting to show whether the change is achieving its objective?

(2) Has this change indicated the need for other changes?

Implementing change depends very much on the personal style of the manager but managers who successfully achieve change tend to have certain characteristics. These include:

Interest in their own personal development, and the growth of their organisations.

Enthusiasm for change.

Desire for new experiences.

Willingness to take reasonable risks.

Openness to more than one course of action.

Concern for achievement and interesting work.

A somewhat unconventional approach to life.

Willingness to accept others as experts.

More inclined to examine current evidence than rely on past experience.

Concern for human relations as well as efficiency.

A planning and problem-solving approach.

Open, participative relationships with other people.

There are a number of techniques which can be considered in implementing change:

(a) *Unfreeze – Change – Freeze*

Existing ways of doing things are often firmly established, and it is necessary to 'unfreeze' them by discussing them openly, critically examining them, experimenting with new approaches, and seeking new ideas from outside the situation. In this way, weaknesses in current arrangements can be more widely recognised, and people involved will be more inclined to accept changes. As change is introduced, new policies and procedures are made and these are then 'frozen' to become part of the new way of doing things.

(b) *Change agent*

Usually it is the 'manager' who is the 'change agent' but often it can be useful to involve an outside person or agency to help bring about change. For example, if a new approach to family planning is being introduced, it can be helpful to bring in the expertise of someone who is regularly involved in the new approach and knows what problems may be encountered. Such a person could be very helpful in giving advice, and helping local workers to understand what is involved, but the local manager cannot leave the whole task of introducing change to an outsider – the local manager still retains responsibility for managing the change.

(c) *A planning approach to management*

A management team which adopts a planning approach to its work will be committed to 'change' as a normal part of its work. Aims and objectives will be regularly reviewed, problems identified, solutions proposed, and action plans worked out. As action plans are regularly used and put into practice, it will be recognised that change is a normal feature of working life.

(d) *Force Field analysis*

An analysis of what is involved in a change by specifying clearly the change which is to be made, the people who will be involved, and other significant factors. A list is then made of all those factors which are *for* the change (the helping factors), and another list of the factors which are *against* the change (the restraining factors). A manager's task is then to encourage and develop the factors which are operating in favour of the change, and to find ways of counteracting or minimising the factors which work against the change.

Table 5.6 is an analysis of what is involved in establishing a sub-centre to serve a population of 10 000 people.

After the Force Field Analysis of impeding and supporting factors, a check list for organisational change can be helpful when introducing a specific change.

Check list for organisational change

Organisational change is imposed by sudden changes of policy, or slowly evolved by one's department or begun at one's own initiative. But however it arises it can seem threatening to the staff and it will place great responsibilities on the shoulders of the manager. The following questions need to be raised:

How will it look to the staff?

What one sees as a new system, the staff will see as upsetting existing arrangements, creating a lot of transitional chaos and burdens of re-learning for them.

Who is going to be affected by the change – and who else?

The district is a closely-knit system and changes may affect a number of people.

How is it going to affect their work?

Give them more *or* less responsibility?
Make them feel more *or* less of a contributor to the whole district?

Table 5.6 Force Field Analysis for establishing a sub-centre (A systematic approach to looking before we leap! Forces impeding and favouring the objective)

Problem	Establishing a Level B station to serve 10 000 people

Step I	Specification of personnel, selection of village, accommodation, transport

How many staff, what sort of staff (criteria)?
Who will provide accommodation (for the facility and staff housing)?
Criteria for selection of village (size, accessibility, water, communications, health problems of the catchment area, etc.)
Type of transport.
Finance.

Step II People involved

People	Role	Relation to District Health Management Team (DHMT)
Village Dev. Committee and Chief	Finding accommodation. Permission to start.	Link between DHMT and community
District Health Management Team	Supervision, training	–
District Education + Agriculture + Water and Social Welfare Officers	Support, advice and co-operation	Link to local government
Reg. Med. Officer and Nursing Officer	Provision of Level B workers, finance	Link to Ministry
Planning Unit	Training, Level C	Training, planning, advice

Step III Other significant factors

Present post, Level B worker
Personal interest toward work
Attractiveness of post
Basic and social amenities
Interest of community toward Level B

Step IV Restraining and helping factors

Restraining factors	Helping factors
Conflicts in Level B between curative and supervisory (outreach tasks)	Wish for professional health workers in the village
Cultural obstacles (such as objection to bicycles)	Working in a team is more attractive than working alone
Different expectations between community, Level B and DHMT	Living near work place
Lack of basic and social amenities	Personal contacts can give high job satisfaction

Give them a greater *or* smaller sense of achievement?
Make jobs more interesting and complete *or* more fragmentary and unrelated?
Make existing skills more *or* less useful?
Place heavy demands *or* no demands on learning new skills?

How is it going to affect relationships?

Will new groups be formed and existing ones dissolved?
Will any individual become or feel isolated?
Will some good jobs be created which change the status structure of the District?
Will it affect people's lives outside the work situation?

Has enough time been allowed for the following?

Discussion with other managers?
Discussion with staff?
Replanning the whole thing if one needs to in the light of these discussions?

Is a 'third party' involved?

Occasionally consultants and specialists assist such changes. One should try:

To understand their terms of reference clearly.
To ensure that these are known and explained and accepted by the staff involved.
To set up working teams with the specialists – not isolate them.
To remember that their intrusion is commonly resented and one must try not to let such resentment influence one's behaviour.

MANAGING CONFLICTS

In the management of health care conflicts and differences of opinion are inevitable. To give just a few examples – because money is short, health managers will frequently be in discussion with government or other funding agencies to obtain more, and will be in competition with other departments for funds. There will be differences of view within Health Districts on priorities – which diseases should be dealth with first, which village should have more facilities. Workers themselves will have differences – over their pay and conditions of work, working arrangements, and so on. In the Health Team itself there may well be differences on such things as the importance to be given to preventive or curative medicine and the roles of health workers, for example, nurses, medical assistants. The Health Team which is committed to rapid development of Primary Health Care is likely to find that a good deal of its time is spent in dealing with conflicts and reconciling different points of view.

A number of methods may be utilised to manage conflicts as follows:

The problem-solving approach

The basis of this approach is that the best solution to a problem is one that is agreed by all the parties who are affected by the problem. It only works, however, where there is common agreement on the fundamental aims of the group. For example, if there is disagreement in a Health Centre over the allocation of rooms and times for different clinics, those involved can probably discuss the issue and resolve it provided there is general agreement on the over-all aims and priorities for the Health Centre. Where there is fundamental disagreement on the policy for the Health Centre, however, it is unlikely that any amount of discussion will provide a solution. This is why it is important to have agreed aims which are accepted and well understood throughout a Health District. Given such aims, the vast majority of problems can be dealt with through rational discussion and argument. In a problem-solving approach the group concerned goes through the steps of problem solving just as a manager would if he were solving the problems on his own, namely: defining the problem clearly, setting clear objectives for solving the problem, analysing the problem to determine causes and effects, searching for alternative solutions, deciding on the solution which best meets the objectives and agreeing the specific action to be taken.

The benefits of a problem-solving approach are that it can strengthen the involvement and commitment of all those concerned, it can channel people's energies away from destructive conflict towards a constructive search for solutions and it can be a valuable way of generating new ideas and approaches.

Bargaining

This takes place when two parties who are in dispute do not share common aims. There is a large element of bargaining involved in local purchasing, and local personnel may be highly skilled and enjoy the processes of making offers, counter-offers and 'walk-aways' to obtain goods at the lowest possible prices. At a higher organisational level, hard bargaining is called for in deciding expenditure between hospital care and community health. Another example is that of negotiations with drug companies and other suppliers to ensure the supply of the right goods, at the right time, in the right place and at a reasonable cost.

Use of 'third parties'

Where two parties are in dispute, a third party is sometimes called in to settle the issue. Frequently a manager is put in this position when two or more members of staff are unable to agree on an important matter. The manager has the managerial authority to decide one way or the other, according to what is best for the district, and often that decision will be accepted by the parties concerned. But there are times when it is better for the manager not to *arbitrate* and make the decision, but to *conciliate*, that is, to bring the disputing parties together and guide the discussion so that the parties are forced to sort the problem out for themselves.

Avoiding or ignoring the conflict

Managers may pretend that conflict does not exist because they are not sure how to deal with it, or are afraid the conflict may get worse if they get too involved. Unfortunately, unresolved conflicts often tend to get worse. Managers therefore need to be constantly 'listening' for the first signs of major difficulties so that conflicts can be dealt with sooner rather than later. It helps to recognise that differences of opinion and interest are an inevitable part of the management task. Effective managers are skilled in dealing with differences and recognise some of their positive side-effects. Differences can be used as a means of generating new ideas and approaches, through the use of problem-solving discussions to resolve difficulties. Through facing up to the realities of power and individual interest, managers learn how to advance the cause of improved health for the community, and how to win the support of powerful interest groups. And by successfully resolving conflicts, managers are able to build up strong relationships with both health workers and others in the community.

GIVING SUPPORT TO SUPERVISORS

The job of a supervisor is both responsible and difficult. Supervisors frequently have had little formal training in supervision, work in geographical isolation, and tackle all the problems of organising work and supervising staff in the most difficult circumstances. Managers who can give good support to supervisors will find that it results in the improved quality of health services.

Generally, supervisors become so through promotion, because they have been good workers themselves. This can be a great strength in that the supervisor knows thoroughly the work which has to be done, the practical problems and how to get over them. The supervisor is also likely to have a close affinity with other workers, often coming from the same social background, speaking the same language, and sharing a common approach to life. But ability to do a job well does not automatically make someone a good supervisor of other people.

The job of supervisors

There are certain elements which are frequently found in the work of supervisors, which include the following:
    (1) To plan the work of the department/section/health facility.
    (2) To allocate work to individuals.
    (3) To co-ordinate the work of different people.
    (4) To see that work is done to a proper standard.
    (5) To communicate
        (a) to workers – aims and objectives, work to be done, changes, and so on;
        (b) to managers – reports, needs, difficulties.
    (6) To demonstrate, train, support, help and encourage workers to do their work well.
    (7) To solve workers' problems when needed.
    (8) To improve working methods.
    (9) To maintain healthy and safe premises and working methods.
  (10) To ensure a good working environment – physically and socially.
  (11) To act as the level of policy-making closest to workers.

The supervisor should be well aware that to do the job well certain supervisory 'tools' are needed. These are akin to 'tools of the trade' which a craftsman or other workers would use and include such things as:

Schedules/Timetables/Diaries/Programmes – because much of a supervisor's work consists of getting certain things done at certain times (for example, clinic sessions, supplies requisitions, visiting programmes, and so on), a systematic way of planning and controlling such activities is needed.
Instruction guides and procedures – to help with work which is of a semi-routine or systematic nature, for example, procedures for weighing and examination under-fives, diagnosing and treating common complaints, reviewing activities of the village health workers and so on.
Rules and regulations – these should be simple and clear to understand. Out-of-date and complicated regulations can be more of a hindrance than a help.
Budgets – this refers usually to money which can be spent within a set period of time. For the supervisor a more tangible set of budgets is needed, for example, numbers of staff and working hours available for certain tasks; amounts of overtime or extra payments which may be authorised; amounts

of drugs, vaccines and other supplies available per month; mileage and travelling allowances per month. These are budgets which a supervisor should account for in some detail and exercise close control over.

Support for supervisors

Above all supervisors need support from their own 'supervisors' or managers and this should include:

Leadership in the form of clear guidance from their own manager when needed; trust, and regular contact.

Training in preparation and on appointment as a supervisor; and as a continuing process, both on and off the job. Because of the practical nature of the work, supervisors can gain much by discussing with other supervisors various aspects of their jobs.

Backing for decisions. Supervisors must know that they will get support whenever they have to make decisions within their own sphere of responsibility. Even where bad decisions are made, it is important that supervisors receive support especially in the eyes of their own staff, whilst being given help to redress the situation and guidance on how to make better decisions in the future. It is better for the occasional mistake to be made than for supervisors to be afraid of making any decision.

Recognition and proper status for the supervisor's own position. This means that a manager should not try to 'by-pass' the supervisor in dealing with members of staff, and as much as possible should work with the supervisor in explaining and discussing future plans, changes, and so on, with staff.

Reliability. Despite the many problems involved, supervisors should be able to rely on supplies of drugs and other materials arriving when expected; a regular pattern of visits from their managers; and above all action promised by managers should in fact be taken.

Involvement in planning. Because supervisors are nearest to the 'grass roots' of the health service, they have an important contribution to make in planning for the future. Through sharing in planning, supervisors can develop a broader outlook on the task of health provision and further their own personal development to take on increased managerial responsibility in the future.

PERSONNEL – THE MANAGEMENT OF HEALTH WORKERS

Rural health services rely on the efficiency and enthusiasm of the staff who run them. 'Personnel Management' is the aspect of management which ensures that everything concerned with the employment of staff within the Health District is done effectively, so that staff can be happy in their work and give of their best. Much of the job of personnel management is done by managers within the District such as the District Medical Officer, Head of Nursing, Heads of Health Centres and so on. But other important aspects of personnel management (for example, establishment of personnel policies and procedures, negotiation and payment of salaries and wages, the running of training schemes) may be carried out centrally, at District, Regional or National level. Many personnel practices may be already established in a well-run hospital, and the task of the District Medical Officer may be to ensure that these practices apply within the rural sector of the District. In other cases existing personnel policies and practices may need to be adapted for the Primary Health Sector.

The management of health workers includes:

Recruitment and selection – searching for and choosing workers for particular posts. By taking the trouble to select good workers, many problems can be avoided and a high quality of work achieved.

Induction and training – ensuring that new workers are properly introduced to their work, and continue to be trained to do their work well.

Allocating work –giving workers tasks which are within their capabilities and make the best use of their skills and knowledge.

Supervision – ensuring that workers can always get help when they need it and that high standards of work are maintained.

Discipline and grievance – Dealing effectively but fairly with workers who break rules or whose work is not up to standard; and settling speedily any grievances or disputes which workers themselves may have.

Good communications – ensuring that there is two-way open communication between workers, their supervisors and members of the Health Team.

Counselling and guidance – helping workers to solve day-to-day difficulties, or personal problems which affect their work.

Promotion and career development – giving workers the chance to 'better themselves' whilst ensuring a supply of workers who can take on more responsibility in the future.

Manpower planning

Manpower planning is concerned with 'team-building' for the future. Managers need to consider future staffing needs, existing and potential sources of supply, recruitment, training and development strategies to ensure that trained staff will be available to do the work called for in the District's long-term plans.

In most countries recruitment and selection of staff occurs centrally at the National level and the District Medical Officer will find his staff appointed by a distant Ministry of Health. Many of them may be recent graduates with little experience. Here the challenge is to mould the various workers into a team and to identify from amongst the team members those who show promise for future promotion to positions of responsibility. As an aid to selection a technique which has been widely adopted is that of the 'seven-point plan'. This is a means of considering the factors which should appear in a personnel specification under seven main headings, as follows:

Physical make-up

Are there any important defects of health or physique? How important are appearance, bearing and speech?

Attainments

What level of education and training, occupational training and experience is needed?

General intelligence

What level of intelligence is needed? Intelligence is not always related to education!

Special aptitudes

Is there a need for any special skills? Facility in the use of words? Or figures? Any unusual talents?

Interests

Are these intellectual? Practical? Physical? Social? Artistic? and so on.

Disposition

For example, acceptability to other people. Ability to influence others? Dependability. Self-reliance.

Circumstances

Family responsibilities, housing needs, and so on. What do other members of the family do for a living? Are there any special openings available?

The aim of the Seven-Point Plan is to try to obtain as complete and objective a picture of the candidate as possible. It can reduce the subjective element in selection, and act as a frame of reference in comparing one person with another. It also provides a systematic framework for asking questions of candidates and carrying out an effective interview.

In appointing staff to various positions it will help to have a full description of the job the individual is expected to do. This will help in 'fitting' the most suitable person to a job. Moreover, the process of writing a job description entails job analysis which provides an insight into what is expected and required in the job. In turn this helps with job evaluation, work organisation and review of the candidate's performance. The exercise may also raise questions of training, and any deficiency can be rectified through in-service training programmes. These various inter-relationships are shown diagramatically in figure 4.7 (p. 112).

TRAINING

Rural health services largely depend on auxiliary health personnel. The rural health organisation has been described as a 'skill pyramid' in which skills in health care are widely distributed amongst those who provide health services, and not restricted to doctors and nurses who have had intensive medical and clinical training. Training needs to be 'built in' as part of the normal activity of the district, and not seen solely as something which takes place in training schools or is 'added on' to the normal working routine when there is time to do it.

There needs to be a *present* and a *future* orientation to the way in which people's work is viewed. Staff need training to carry out their existing work competently but they also need to learn how to achieve higher levels of competence in the future, either within their existing work, or by promotion to a job with greater responsibilities. There needs then to be a *training plan* for every worker in the health district. It is unlikely that this will always be written down (though there is merit in writing it down annually for each *senior* member of staff), but each worker and his supervisor should have a clear idea of which aspects of the work they are currently learning to improve and which new skills they are developing. Ideally every team leader or supervisor should have a Training Plan for their own unit indicating who needs to learn what and how urgently. The most important Training Plan in the District is that of the District Medical Officer himself. Table 5.7 indicates what such a Training Plan

Table 5.7 **Example of a training plan**

Training plan   Dr...............   D.M.O...............   District.............

	Supervisory Skills							'Technical' Skills					Management Skills				'Broadening' Skills			
	Giving instructions and training	Dealing with staff's problems	Communication	Allocating and organising work	Dealing with sub-standard work	Support to village health workers	Team leadership	Drug prescribing	Referrals	Health education	Treatment	Diagnosis	Information for evaluation	Financial control	Managing drugs & supplies	Forward planning	Improved clinical knowledge	Wider management skills	Understanding of community	Other aspects of health care
Mr A. Health Centre Supervisor	B	B	A	A	B	B	C													
Mrs B. Health Centre Head Nurse	B	A	A	C	A	A	B													
Mrs C Health Centre Public Health Nurse	C	B	B	B	A	A	A													
Miss D. Community Midwife	A	C	A	B	A	B	B	MCH Organisation A B B												
Mr E. Chief Sanitarian								Appropriate technology for: (a) water –A (b) sanitation –B												

Key: C = Competent
      B = Needs improvement
      A = Needs major improvement

might look like, and obviously would need to be adapted to local circumstances, but it can give managers some basis for organising training.

It is clear that the type of training suggested is not of the 'recent advances' or 'update' kind, but practical training related to the day-to-day work of the individual. Besides the training plan, resources need to be made available. Time and money spent on training is not a misuse of resources but can lead to large 'pay-offs' in the future. Health workers need to see their work as a training task – the population being taught how to maintain its own health, and workers learning how to carry out increased responsibilities. If this attitude is prevalent then many working situations can be used as training opportunities.

Staff training will fall into the following categories:

New health workers – induction training to acquaint them with their responsibilities and local circumstances.

Staff about to take on new responsibilities.

'Students' (for example, trainee community nurses) attached for practical training.

Those whose work is not up to standard.

Those who need refresher training, for example, community health workers, traditional birth attendants, and so on.

STAFF DEVELOPMENT

Just as Management Teams make plans to improve health services, so they should also plan the development needs of workers. Individuals should be helped to improve their skills and qualifications and move on to posts of greater responsibility. Many bright young people who get some education in the rural areas leave for the towns because they see the urban market as the only way of realising their ambitions and aspirations. It should be possible to retain a number of these people if the Health Care system offers the right kind of opportunities. Positive policies for staff development in the District should include:

(a) *Selection policies.* As far as possible workers should come from the village or district being served. Workers should be acceptable to the local community, but those with education and initiative should be encouraged to take on more responsibility in the future.

(b) *Promotion.* First consideration should be given to people already working in the health district. This does not mean appointing people who are not properly qualified, but that training and developing of staff is a major responsibility of the District Health Manager.

(c) *Future opportunities.* There should be realistic opportunities for those with initiative, and workers should be able to see how they can progress to more responsible work. Lack of basic education will be a bar to many positions, and opportunities need to be created for the training and advancement of those with little or no basic education.

(d) *Links with training institutions* both within and outside the district. Qualified nurses are likely to be trained at a Regional or 'Teaching' hospital, medical assistants may be trained at a Regional Centre. An 'active' District will be looking for candidates for these posts from the District and the local community, encouraging the training schools to use the District for field attachments, providing 'vacation' work opportunities where appropriate, and encouraging students to return to the District after training. It could be the personal responsibility of a District Medical Officer to seek out and maintain links with medical students who have been 'on attachment' or spent 'elective periods' in the District and who might ultimately return to work as an assistant!

(e) *Good internal training in the District.* To ensure competent workers who are able to take on more responsibility in the future.

(f) *Regular appraisal.* The opportunity for more senior staff (for example, Health Centre Supervisors) to meet with their senior manager specifically to talk about their own work performance, how it might be improved, and what can be done about their own personal development.

(g) *Opportunities at the District level of health care.* There may be openings for Primary Health Care staff in the District Hospital, which can help hospital staff to have a better understanding of the needs of the wider community.

(h) *Flexibility.* A narrow 'professionalism' has constantly to be fought. For example, doctors, nurses, sanitary inspectors or health assistants jealously guard their own particular expertise and refuse to share it with others, or allow others to do work which traditionally they have regarded as their own. The more a number of workers exist who can step into another's role, the more each worker benefits and is equipped for broader responsibilities in the future.

(i) *Support for educational opportunities.* Close links with primary and secondary schools can ensure that Health Education and health matters are dealt with in the schools, but also can ensure that workers get help with their own education. Active involvement in such activities as the 'Child to Child' programme, adult education classes, and distance teaching by radio programmes can lead to continuing improvement in general education for health workers.

(j) *Balance between educated and experienced workers.* As educational opportunities improve there are dangers that better educated, younger people come in to take all the interesting, responsible work and block off opportunities for hard working, conscientious but less well-educated workers who normally advance through the ranks by accumulating experience. It is very important to be sensitive to the problems this can cause and ensure that there is a proper balance between workers and opportunities to which all can aspire.

(k) *Coaching.* This implies the conscious, systematic and regular effort to learn from normal work activities. People often learn best from what they find out for themselves. So a District Medical Officer on regular visits to a Health Centre Supervisor can guide, explain and assign more challenging tasks from which the supervisor can 'learn by doing.'

(l) *Local study days.* There may be transport problems to be overcome, but the effort may be well worthwhile of arranging for health workers from right across a District to come together to listen to a special speaker, for example, a Regional Agricultural Officer, or Regional Medical Officer, or to see some new technique, simple equipment or teaching aid. Such a day also provides the opportunity to consider how new ideas and approaches can be implemented throughout a District.

The above suggestions indicate a wide range of activities which can improve the development of staff in a district. There may not be time to engage in all of them simultaneously, but the key is to start on some of them. Staff development activities can require a lot of attention in the first instance, but once under way, can grow and multiply with workers taking more and more initiative for their own development. The fundamental requirement is an attitude of mind that development of staff is essential for better performance and improvement of services.

MAINTAINING STANDARDS AND DISCIPLINE

Those in managerial and leadership positions need to have high standards for their own work, and maintain similar high standards throughout the organisation. Where high standards are set and achieved, and where workers know what standard of work is expected of them, it should rarely be necessary to take disciplinary action against any worker provided care has been taken in the selection and training of the workers and they are given support and supervision. However, there are occasions when someone's work does not come up to expectation and disciplinary action has to be taken. For such occasions disciplinary rules and procedures are needed which are understood, and accepted as fair and reasonable.

Disciplinary rules should define the minimum standards of behaviour at work like, for example, work performance standards, requirements to obey reasonable instructions and the prescribed punishment for serious misconduct.

A disciplinary procedure sets out action to be taken when rules are broken or work is unsatisfactory. Procedures enable managers to deal effectively with the situation, and deal fairly with the worker concerned. Disciplinary procedures should:

(1) Be in writing.
(2) Specify to which grades of staff they apply (for example, there may be different procedures for professional staff and less skilled workers).
(3) Provide for speedy operation.
(4) State the range of disciplinary actions that can be taken (for example, dismissal, suspension with or without pay, reprimand, transfer).
(5) Specify those who have authority to take action (for example, a procedure may state that a Health Centre Supervisor has authority to reprimand but not to dismiss).
(6) Provide for investigation before disciplinary action is taken. Where the rules provide for instant dismissal (for example, for serious misconduct) the first step may need to be suspension while the case is investigated. An action taken in the heat of the moment may cause difficulties later.
(7) Ensure that individuals are informed of any complaint and given opportunity to state their case.
(8) Give an individual the right to be accompanied by a representative or friend.
(9) Ensure that reasons are given for any penalty imposed.
(10) Give a right of appeal if individuals feel they have been unfairly treated. This appeal may be to a higher level of management, or where appropriate to a village committee or a local leader in the case of a village health worker.
(11) Give individuals the opportunity to improve their conduct after a first warning.
(12) Provide for one or more warnings (depending on the seriousness of the offence).
(13) Ensure that authority to dismiss does not rest with a worker's immediate supervisor, but with a more senior person. Dismissal should normally only occur where repeated warnings have been ignored or there is gross misconduct.
(14) Provide for dismissal if an offence is repeated after a final warning.
(15) Ensure that all workers know what rules and procedures apply to

them, and that managers and supervisors also clearly understand the part they have to play.

In a number of countries employment legislation requires employers to deal reasonably with employees in disciplinary matters. Such legislation should not make it harder to discipline or dismiss unsatisfactory workers. With clearly understood rules and procedures both managers and workers know where they stand, and if disciplinary action is needed, it can be dealt with in a reasonable and straightforward manner. Even with well-understood rules and procedures, the most important factors in maintaining high standards of work and discipline are the standards which managers and supervisors set for themselves, and the quality of support and supervision they give to their workers.

COUNSELLING – OR HELPING STAFF WITH THEIR PROBLEMS

'Counselling' is an important part of the job for many health workers. For example, a public health nurse will 'counsel' or discuss with a mother those personal and family problems which affect the growth and development of her baby. But health workers themselves have problems of their own which may be personal or related to work, and managers are often asked for help and advice.

So much of the Health Manager's task consists of supporting, guiding, and helping other people to do things well that it is worth looking at some of the helping, 'counselling' relationships. The danger is that managers often feel that they know best how to offer solutions whereas what is important is that workers need to be helped to define their own problems, clarify and explore them, and try to find realistic solutions. It is obvious that managers need to be good at listening and at encouraging workers with a problem to express their feelings about it. This requires a high degree of concentration and the ability to observe what the worker is trying to say. Communication between individuals can be difficult because of personal, psychological and sociological differences. These can be accentuated when the manager has a different regional, ethnic and language background, a higher 'professional' status, and little knowledge of the details of someone's day-to-day life and work.

Some managers feel happier with a 'directive' and others with a 'non-directive' approach to counselling. In the directive approach the manager will give clear direction and advice. In non-directive counselling the manager does not suggest solutions but helps workers solve their own problems. There are situations which call for a 'directive' approach, for example where standards of work have to be maintained; but the effective manager is the one who can adopt a 'directive' or 'non-directive' approach depending on the circumstances.

FINANCE

Managers need to ensure that Primary Health Care actually gets all the financial support that is available to it and that money does not get siphoned off into hospitals; is used effectively and is not wasted either fraudulently or through inefficiency, and is available for future as well as present needs. To meet such needs various financial techniques and systems have been developed. The best systems are often the simplest, but the important thing is that the Health Management Team must work closely with their financial colleagues, share an understanding of each other's functions, and develop practical systems which effectively meet their needs.

Although the development of Primary Health Care (PHC) may be stipulated in a District Development Plan, the implementation of that plan will be highly dependent on the finance available. If for any reason, for example, inflation, economic recession, political changes, those allocations are reduced, there will be a danger of the PHC programme being cut back to ensure the continuance of hospital services. Moreover, there is a natural tendency for the financial demands of the hospital to grow. Spending patterns and proposals in the hospital should therefore be critically examined to ensure that they do not lead to further imbalances between primary and secondary care.

Sources of finance

Sources of finance should be clearly identified, and the best possible case put forward for obtaining a satisfactory allocation. Hospital services have often developed faster than primary care because hospital doctors and managers have been highly skilled at putting forward the case for finance to develop those services. As governments increasingly provide the main funds for health services, a clear understanding of how government funding arrangements operate is needed.

Other non-governmental sources of income should not be neglected. Grants from aid and development agencies, missions, and so on, can be important sources of finance, perhaps related to individual or special projects, often of an innovative or enterprising nature. The key to securing or maintaining such grants depends on the strength and clarity of the case put forward. The case should include (a) a specification of the *goals* to be achieved (for example, a

nutrition project, immunisation programme, establishment of a health post),
(b) details of the *action plan* (milestones) proposed to achieve the goals, (c)
identification of the *resources* needed (for example, initial expenses, building,
equipment, and so on, and operating expenses – staff, supplies, and so on), and
(d) an outline *budget* showing how much finance is needed for each year of the
project for each item of expense. Much of this information will be included
in the District Plan. Moreover, help is usually available from aid agencies
which normally provide details of what information is needed and how to
present it.

An important part of the Primary Health Care concept is that as far as
possible local communities should support their own health services. In some
places fees for services, for example, attendances at health centres and medical
consultations, are charged for those who can afford it; in others, villages may
raise levies (for example, on agricultural produce at the time of sale) to help
pay for health services, or may support village health workers in cash or in
kind. Charges may also be made for supplies of drugs, nutritional supplements, contraceptive devices and so on. There is a delicate balance to be
maintained in raising finance locally. On the one hand, it can be good for
people to contribute to their own health services because a service that is paid
for is often valued and appreciated and put to good use. There can also be a
greater sense of involvement where money is raised locally and used on local
projects, rather than raised through taxation and channelled back into health
services through central government funding. On the other hand, when
charges are made there is the very real danger that those who most need health
services will not get them because they cannot afford them; also that the most
beneficial and cost-effective services for example, preventive or environmental
health services will not be financed because they are usually not felt to be
important, and cannot be paid for through individual charges. Resentment
may also build up where local people who are already paying high taxes
without seeing any benefit to themselves are asked to finance their own health
services. In addition, when local charges are made, the administrative costs of
collection, coupled with the hazards of fraud and misappropriation, can
outweigh the benefits of the funds actually raised.

Health Care Plans and Programmes need to be translated into *financial
plans* concerned with estimated capital and revenue expenditure for both the
longer-term Strategic Plan and the shorter-term Operational Plan. As capital
expenditure is concerned with expensive items of buildings or equipment, the
expenditure is often spread over a number of years and can be shown in the
form of a *capital plan*.

A *revenue plan* relates to the day-to-day running of services. The financial
plan should show the amounts allocated for the current year, as well as for future
years. Estimates and forecasts for future years need to take into account
inflation and proposed changes in the levels of services to be provided and
income expected.

Operating Budgets

Capital and revenue plans show the future plans for the District expressed in financial terms over a number of years. Operating budgets are concerned with the application of that plan for the current year. The first step is to obtain a more precise estimate of income and expenditure for the coming year. The predictions in the financial plan need to be reassessed in the light of income and expenditure in the previous year, and a new budget prepared.

It is a good principle of management that budgets should be held at as low a level in the organisation as practicable, so as to give those who actually use resources of money, staff, supplies, and so on, the responsibility for controlling them and using them effectively. The District Health Team should have over-all control of the District Health Budget, with individual managers accountable for parts of it, for example, the District Nursing Officer controlling the nursing budget. Once a budgeting system is established and working well, greater responsibility for budget control can be given to those more closely involved in the day to day provision of health services. This is done by establishing 'budget centres', for example, individual Health Centres, a mobile team, primary health services based at the District Hospital, and so on. The appropriate 'manager', for example, the Health Centre Supervisor or leader of the mobile team as the case may be, is involved in preparing, controlling and managing that part of the budget, whilst members of the District Health Team retain over-all budget responsibility.

Budgets offer an effective means of planning, implementation and evaluation. When budgets are prepared with desired outcomes or utilities in view, the process can be referred to as programmed budgeting. Money is allocated to specific programmes within the District Health Plan, for example, to health education, family planning, immunisation, rather than to 'lines', that is, furniture, refrigerators, equipment and so on. Programme budgeting allows health programmes to be viewed as part of an over-all health plan designed to achieve defined and measurable objectives of the whole health plan of the district.

The allocation of funds to programmes must be done in such a way that the programmes likely to contribute more substantially to the realisation of the aims and objectives of the District Health Plans are weighted. This enables scarce funds to be distributed more rationally. For programme budgets to be costed accurately and uniformly, 'standard cost lists' provided for various economic zones of the whole country by an appropriate government agency can be very helpful. Such 'standard cost lists' contain information on salaries and allowances for professional and other health workers and costs of standard equipment, vehicles and spare parts, and so on.

Programme planning and budgeting is a useful technique because it compels District health staff, indeed all health staff, to plan carefully their health activities and set well-defined and measurable objectives. This way the District budget becomes a management tool which can provide the feedback (evaluation) necessary for the redefining of objectives should this be necessary.

Costing information

Relevant costing information can help a District Health Team in its management task. A number of questions come to mind: Which are the most expensive health centres to run in the District? Which are the least expensive? What is the cost of treating a particular condition with Drug A as opposed to Drug B? What is the cost of running Mother and Child Health Clinics in different parts of the District? What is the cost of running such clinics with fully trained as compared with less well-trained workers? What are the cost implications of alternative health care strategies?

Costing is the process of bringing together all the costs associated with a particular aspect of the health services (for example, a Health Centre and its outlying village services; a District's sanitation or environmental health programme; a training school for health auxiliaries; a specific immunisation programme) in order to assess what it actually costs to provide that service. Costing information is needed to assess the feasibility of new programmes or services; to assess whether services are becoming more or less expensive; to make cost comparisons between different programmes and facilities (for example, different Health Centres); and to provide control information for Government or other funding agencies.

Key elements in costing include:

(a) Identifying 'Cost Centres' – for example, Health Centre X, Malaria control, Vaccination programme, and so on.
(b) Allocating costs, including direct and indirect costs, to the Cost Centre
   (i) Direct costs – costs directly affecting the Cost Centre, for example, salary of Health Centre Superintendent, cost of malaria control.
   (ii) Indirect costs – Costs 'shared' by the Cost Centre with other cost centres. For example, a proportion of the cost of the DMOH (salary, and so on) as part of the DMOH's time is spent in supporting the work of the Health Centre or programme.
(c) Quantification of 'units of service' provided for example, numbers of patients seen in a health centre or clinic, numbers of vaccinations given.
(d) Cost ratios. A combination of (b) and (c) which shows the cost of a particular unit of service, for example,

$$\frac{\text{Total costs of vaccination programme in one year}}{\text{Numbers of people vaccinated}} = \text{Cost per vaccination}$$

This simple 'cost per person vaccinated' can then be used to assess the value of a particular vaccination programme, to determine charges, or to make cost comparisons between different vaccination programmes.

Financial reports

In addition to reports and statements concerned with Planning, Budgeting, Cost Control, and so on, there are other documents, for example, Balance Sheet, Income and Expenditure Statements, Statistical Reports, which are prepared from time to time by accountants and finance departments. It can be very valuable for a District Health Team to have some insight into the purpose served by such documents and what additional information can be derived from them, as an aid to a better understanding of the financial 'health' of a district. A useful question to have in mind is: 'If this were my money that was being spent, what information and checks would I want to have to be sure that my money was being used properly?'.

BUILDINGS

Buildings in the form of dispensaries, Health Centres, clinics and hospitals are part of the normal set-up for health care. There are, however, advantages *and* disadvantages in relying on buildings as a principal means of providing health care (see table 5.8).

Managers need to think very carefully before deciding to spend money on new buildings or on the extension of existing ones. A first consideration should always be: How can a health plan be developed which makes the minimum use of buildings? A survey should also be made of buildings and facilities already in the community in which health services could be provided or developed, for example,

schools – development of child health services
    – use during or outside normal school hours
missions, religious premises – may have room or under-used capacity
    which could be used for clinics, health education activities
houses, homes – of village health workers, local healers or others can be
    adapted or extended for health purposes
village meeting places, community development, agriculture projects – may
    all have useful facilities
commercial premises – private pharmacies and drug stores
workplaces – employers may be encouraged to provide facilities for their
    employees, families and immediate neighbours

Table 5.8 **Buildings for health care**

Advantages	Disadvantages
Provide *privacy* for personal consultations	*Expensive* both to build and maintain
Provide *security* for equipment, stores, drugs, etc.	*Distant* from many homes in the community
Provide *shelter* from rain, heat etc.	Tend to serve only the *immediate locality*
Enable facilities and resources to be *concentrated* in one place	*Isolate* staff from the community they are meant to serve
Are a *visible focus* for health care	Become an *end in themselves* rather than a means to better health
Are part of the *community* and attract local support	By their existence *separate health* from other aspects of life
Can be *silent teachers* of a clean, hygienic way of life	Encourage institutional thinking rather than problem-solving of the community's needs
Maintain *continuity* of health services as people come and go	*Inflexible* – built for one purpose and difficult to change for another
A base for *teamwork*	Can cause *problems* between staff over use of rooms, etc.
Necessary for complicated medical treatments and procedures	Encourage the use of expensive treatments and procedures

By encouraging local people to extend and make use of such facilities, the community can be encouraged to think of health provision as its own responsibility, and it is also a means of strengthening links between health and other aspects of the community's life.

An assessment should also be made of existing health buildings. A worrying feature of health provision in a number of countries is the extent to which buildings put up in the past are not being fully used. Health Centres which were intended to provide a basic range of services may be under-utilised, whilst people travel long distances to overcrowded hospitals to obtain these same services, at much higher cost and inconvenience to themselves and the hospital. Such by-pass phenomena are a challenge to Health Managers and the reasons need to be investigated and put right. Often it has been the case that Health Centres were established but were not adequately staffed or supported; the services they provided therefore were not adequate to begin with and may have deteriorated further; the population lost confidence and no longer went to the Health Centre but went instead to the already crowded hospital. In this situation what is needed are not new buildings, but attention to the management deficiencies at the root of the problem. An assessment of existing buildings should therefore cover the following points:

Usage   are health buildings under-used or over-used?

Activities	what clinics, out-patient, in-patient, teaching activities take place? Should such activities continue? Are they scheduled and organised efficiently?
Size	is the building too big, too small? What can be done about it? Develop new activities? Extend the building?
Location	are buildings most conveniently located for access by the population? Where should any new buildings be placed?
Condition	are repairs needed? Is maintenance being regularly carried out?
Staffing	are there the right numbers and quality of staff? Is suitable training available?
Support	is there sufficient support from the local community and the health service to carry out the function expected?
Supplies	are the supplies of drugs and equipment regular, with adequate stocks of essential drugs?
Facilities/Services	does the building have the necessary furniture, equipment and services (for example, water supply) to do its job effectively?
Security	is the building safe from misuse, theft, and so on?
Flexibility	how easy is it to adapt the building to new purposes?
Operational policies	are there clear statements of how the various activities which take place within the building are to be organised?

The work involved in actually planning, designing and constructing a new health building is a study in its own right and most countries have standard plans for Health Centres, sub-centres and hospitals. A practical guide entitled 'A Model Health Centre', published in 1975 by the Conference of Medical Missionary Societies in Great Britain and Ireland, links the practical and technical aspects of Health Centre building including such aspects as Staffing, Workloads, Social Areas, Room Layouts, Storage Facilities and Record Keeping, and so on.

SUPPLIES AND STORES

An effective supplies system is essential for the smooth running of rural health care. The range of goods and equipment needed is not in itself large, but the confidence that the right goods will be in the right place at the right time is crucial. A Primary Health Care supplies system should be relatively simple and straightforward, and should relate to other supplies systems in the District, for example, public transport; systems based on a District Hospital; or other agencies like Agriculture, Community Development and so on. Greater efficiency and savings can be made by co-ordinating transport and distribution systems in remote and widespread rural areas.

Essentially, a supplies system deals with requisitioning or ordering, purchasing, receipt, care and custody, and finally, issue of goods to users. In most countries the Central Stores Department, advised and guided by a Pharmaceutical Supplies Committee at the Ministry of Health, undertakes these functions and provides a service for the Primary Health Care Programme. The Central Medical Stores at the National level has its branches and counterparts at the Regional and District level. Besides these central supplies, there may be a small allocation for local purchase of drugs not provided by the Central Medical Stores.

A centralised store at District level needs a full-time storekeeper with expertise in supervising the various stages of supplies management. Each village health worker should be issued with a box containing essential drugs, dressings, and so on. Members of the District Health Team must be familiar with the way in which the system operates to ensure that the essential requirements for providing Primary Health Care are in regular supply. Too little held in stock can lead to frequent shortages; large stocks are costly and provide greater opportunity for pilferage, deterioration, over-ordering and other abuses. In determining how much stock to hold the following factors should be taken into account:

Monthly, quarterly or annual requirements for each item
The price of items
The time taken between placing an order and receiving the goods
The purchasing cost for each order

Stores *records* are important. The *inventory* is a list of furniture and equipment for which a manager is responsible in each health building or mobile team. It should be kept up to date and checked regularly to keep control over losses, breakages, stealing, and so on. A *requisition* is an order form for obtaining goods from Central Stores; a good principle of delegation is that the person who uses supplies should have the authority to requisition them subject to supervision by the manager. Within a Central Store, records of goods held in stock will be kept in a *store ledger*, and that should agree with the number of items on the shelves of the store which are also noted on a *tally card* or bin card. As goods are received into the store, entries are made in the ledger and on the tally cards, and as goods are issued against a requisition appropriate entries are also made on a *stores issue voucher* and in a *stores issues book*.

Each health centre should have its strong-room for storage. Clear and well-understood supplies procedures are needed to ensure that goods are ordered and obtained before stocks run down, and a system of periodic stock-taking and auditing to ensure that goods are not lost, stolen, or misappropriated, or deteriorate through poor storage.

Where certain goods are used frequently, for example, dressings, needles, and so on, re-ordering is simplified by having a 'topping-up' system whereby a top limit of, say, 50 or 100 items is held at any one time, and stocks are replenished to this level each time deliveries are made. Control over the use of those items is obtained by setting an upper limit to the number which can be used in any given period of time.

Problems in supplies organisation need to be identified and remedied. *National* shortages cannot be dealt with locally, so what few supplies are available must be used for priority cases, and where possible alternative or locally available supplies used. Where the problem is of *transport* or *distribution* those systems need to be looked at and improvements made. Often shortages at the peripheral level are due to a poor transport and distribution system or inefficient management rather than due to national shortages. Usually problems arise through *inefficiencies* and *over-bureaucratic controls* which need to be dealt with thoroughly. *Over-stocking* and *fraud* need to be tackled immediately. If there is insufficient money available to buy necessary goods and supplies, then *budget allocations* may need to be reviewed. Managers need to develop health care and prevention activities which rely as little as possible on imported expensive supplies and equipment, and to become skilled in using locally available resources and technology for health care purposes.

DRUGS, VACCINES AND OTHER PHARMACEUTICALS

The control and eradication of many diseases in developing countries depends on the systematic and proper use of drugs and vaccines. The cost of drugs can be high, and health managers face pressures both from local populations who see drugs as the solution to their health problems, and from drug companies who wish to extend their sales. In developing countries drugs can contribute to more than 50 per cent of medical costs. At the same time, in many places great savings could be made through changes in prescribing practices. Effective systems are therefore needed to deal with the standardisation, procurement, distribution, use and control of drugs.

Management of any supply system for drugs and pharmaceuticals may be usefully discussed under three main headings: (i) Procurement, (ii) Indenting and (iii) Standardisation, storage and distribution.

Procurement is best done centrally for countries which depend on outside sources of supply. Decentralised procurement is recommended for drugs with a short shelf life or those required for the treatment of relatively uncommon diseases. It is useful if these drugs can be made available at local drug stores and pharmacies. In many cases, drugs will have to be procured from outside the District and supplied through a state-sponsored procurement agency. To ensure that high quality drugs are ordered at reasonable cost, such central procurement agencies must ensure that drugs are obtained from reputable pharmaceutical companies and at bulk-purchase prices under contract agreements.

Indenting for drugs should as far as possible be based on epidemiological information obtained from the records of local health care institutions. Drugs form an important element in the District Health Plan which shows the basic pattern of disease in the District and what measures are planned to deal with it. The drug budget is likely to be best spent on a limited range of inexpensive items from a national formulary or standard list for those health needs which are most widespread, for example, antimalarials, vermifuges, iron and vitamins, antibiotics, anti-tuberculosis and anti-leprosy drugs. The anticipated monthly usage should be worked out for each Health Centre, clinic or health worker, and supply and distribution systems co-ordinated to ensure that the right drugs get to the right place at the right time. Adjustments can be made to the quantities of drugs supplied on a month by month basis in relation to the number of cases dealt with. Drugs can be classified into *fast-moving* and *slow-moving items*. Indents for fast-moving items like antibiotics and antimalarials can be prepared in such a way that adequate monthly stock levels are maintained in local Health Centres, and hospitals as well as at District and Regional drug depots to allow free and uninterrupted flow of supplies from the National to the local level. Where possible a 'topping-up' system may be used.

Standardisation is an essential element in efficient drug management, especially at the periphery of a National Health Care system. The principle of standardisation applies to the design of simple drug formularies for use at local levels of the District health care system, depending on the level of training of staff and on the health problems they face. The use of a simple drug formulary can act as a means of checking over-prescribing and limiting the range of drugs which can be prescribed. This will reduce costs and simplify treatment procedures besides simplifying many problems of centralised buying.

Pre-packing of drugs for Health Centres, health posts, polyclinics and community clinics is a means of simplifying prescribing procedures and also acts as a control measure to check over-prescribing and pilfering.

Vaccines

Vaccines present a special problem within the District Health Service distribution system because they have to be kept at cold temperatures in order to maintain potency. The process of distributing vaccines at a constant low temperature from the point of manufacture to the point of use is called the 'cold chain'. It is a complex process as vaccines are frequently made in one country and used in another. Transport to outlying places must be carefully planned. Refrigerators need proper maintenance and reliable fuel supplies. Health Managers need to be knowledgeable about the cold chain, as detailed in the WHO Expanded Programme on Immunisation, and to review regularly the way the cold chain operates in the District.

TRANSPORT

Transport is an essential part of the communications system of a Health District.

Transport is necessary for:

Supervision and support
Distribution of supplies and drugs
Mobile teams
Public health nurses, sanitarians, health educators, family planning workers, and so on, carrying out their work in the community
Training – to take 'teachers' to 'learners' and vice versa
Patients – when referred to Health Centre or hospital for treatment
Data/Information –from villages, Health Centre, to District HQ
Salaries/Wages – for locally based staff
Visits of District Health Team members throughout the District, to other agencies, regional and provincial centres, and so on.

These needs can be considerable, and with the high costs of vehicles, maintenance and fuel, can consume a large part of a District's health budget. One way out of the difficulty is by organising services in such a way that people at local level do as much as possible for themselves, and do not travel unnecessarily outside their locality. Village health workers, by definition, live within their villages and do not need transport. Health Centres should be based in or near to larger settlements with as good road and path communications as possible. Many members of the outreach team at health centres, for example, community nurses, midwives and so on, may be encouraged to use bicycles. Communication and transport needs in the District should be properly co-ordinated. Thus a weekly or fortnightly return journey by a multi-purpose vehicle between the District HQ and each Health Centre could be used to combine supervision and support, distribution of supplies and drugs, visits of public health nurses and others for specialist clinics, payment of wages, returns of data and information, and for training.

Appropriate resources need to be put into transport. A well-maintained 4-wheel-drive vehicle may be essential to a well-run District, so that contact can always be maintained throughout the community, but other transport needs may be met by simpler means, for example, bicycles, motor cycles, foot or boat and public buses. The principle applying to transport is that simple health care requires simple, not sophisticated support.

As the entire work of the District can break down if the transport system breaks down, likely problems should be identified and ways of dealing with them worked out (see table 5.9)

Table 5.9 **Transport problems and how to tackle them**

Problem	*Ways of tackling the problem*
Breakdown of vehicles	Ensure regular maintenance with log book for each vehicle, showing mileage and type of maintenance required.
	Develop good relationships with local workshops, garages, mechanics.
	Plan for temporary substitution of vehicles, bicycles, and so on.
	Train users in proper upkeep and use of their vehicles.
	Keep a reasonable supply of spares.
	Regular vehicle replacement.
Misuse of vehicles	Good supervision and training.
	Good scheduling of vehicle use, so fewer opportunities for misuse.
	Restrict use to named individuals.
	Effective controls, log-books.
	Enforceable policies on private use.
High transport costs	Examine transport needs – are all journeys really necessary?
	Use low cost transport – bicycles, foot. (A health worker, including doctors and nurses, on a bicycle or on foot gets closer to the community and becomes better known.)
	Standardise vehicles, bicycles and spares.
	Re-examine systems of work in the District.
	Use public transport.
	Work out cost per mile, and transport costs for different services.
	Share transport with other agencies.

FURTHER READING

McGrath, S. J., *Basic managerial skills for all*, Prentice Hall of India Ltd, New Delhi, 1980.

McGregor, D., *The human side of enterprise*, McGraw-Hill, London, 1960.
Stewart, R., *Contrasts in management. A study of the different types of managers jobs: their demands and choices*, McGraw-Hill, London, 1976.
World Health Organization, *Managerial Process for National Health Development: Guiding principles*, WHO, Geneva, 1981.

6 Getting Feedback: Monitoring and Evaluation

Evaluation is a systematic way of learning from experience so as to improve current activities and promote further learning. In the case of health programmes, the objective of evaluation is to improve the services for delivering health care and to guide the allocation of resources. Thus evaluation is closely linked with decision-making both at the operational as well as at policy level.

The same five questions asked about community problems and resources in chapter 2 can be asked about evaluation. Why should we do it? What should be evaluated? How should it be done?, by whom?, where? and when?

WHY DO WE NEED FEEDBACK?

To find out what's going on, to avoid difficulties and problems, and to have information at hand for decisions as they crop up. Getting feedback (or evaluation) is one way of finding out if we are on the right path, and whether health programmes and activities are meeting the needs for which they were drawn up. There is a Ghanaian proverb which says 'If whilst clearing the bush to make a path one does not look back to see where the path is heading in relation to the starting point, one may end up with a path which goes completely round in a circle.' This is why we need feedback about whatever we are doing. This on-going, self-evaluation, is the type of feedback most frequently used in management. It is usually small in scale and short in time. What needs to be monitored is frequently changing depending upon the several activities going on. Information needs to be gathered continually to give an indication of what is happening at the time (see table 6.1).

There are three other forms of evaluation of health care which are frequently

Table 6.1 **Why do we need feedback?**

Type of feedback	Reasons for its use
Assessment of current situation (formative evaluation)	Prior to a project 'Needs assessment' Evaluation of current situation
Assessment of plans (project appraisal)	Are project plans appropriate? – to needs? – to country? – to the people being involved? Political mileage? Blockages for economic reasons?
Intermittent or end of programme (or a particular point in time) (summative evaluation)	Has the project met its long-term objectives? Has the general policy been implemented? Has the donor agency policy been implemented? Shall we continue or discontinue the programme? Shall we replicate the programme elsewhere?
On-going self-evaluation (situational evaluation)	Small-scale, short time period Used by managers and by participating personnel and by communities Must be continually changing and geared directly to short-term action Can improve strategies and techniques

performed and which it is helpful for District Health Teams to know about, even though they may not routinely be involved in them. One type assesses a situation before a project begins. It takes a measure of the existing health services, their utilisation and the health status of the community. It is sometimes called 'needs assessment' or 'formative' evaluation. A second type assesses plans for a project. It is sometimes called 'project appraisal' or 'pre-implementation appraisal'. Programme organisers assess whether a project is appropriate to the identified needs, appropriate to a country and appropriate to the people being involved. This type of evaluation is sometimes vulnerable to people trying to gain political advantage by arguing for a particular type of plan although the country cannot afford it. Alternatively, planners may assume that money is all that matters and may forget they need people who are committed to a plan if it is to be put into action. A third type of evaluation occurs at the end or at a defined stage of a programme or possibly intermittently while the programme is running. It is sometimes called 'summative' evaluation. Its aim is to assess whether a programme has met its long-term objectives, both at a general policy level as well as in detailed outcome measures. It is based on data about outcomes such as morbidity and mortality rates which may only change over long periods of time. Donor agencies often particularly ask for this type of evaluation because it can give a clear idea of what specific gains have been made, and whether their general policy has been put into effect. Finally, all activities and programmes need on-going evaluation by their performers to improve strategies and techniques. All of us concerned with improving the effectiveness of our work are continually doing this but mostly unconsciously or informally. In order to integrate evaluation into the day-to-day work of the manager of the Health Team, it has to be planned for and included in the job description of the manager.

WHAT SHOULD BE EVALUATED?

The next most important question needing an answer is *what* should be evaluated?

What needs to be evaluated depends on the community diagnosis of problems and resources

Community diagnosis (chapter 2) identifies certain problems and potential resources. Evaluation will be able to answer questions such as 'Have the disease problems been altered?' 'What are the new disease problems?' 'Are resources being used effectively?' 'What new resources might be mobilised?' Have the underlying social causes and other determinants of ill health been fully identified? Are the health services well geared to tackle the health problems experienced by the majority of the people in the area?

What needs to be evaluated depends on the plan of action for the health team in the district

The health plan (chapter 3) identified a strategy for action and specific goals and targets. Evaluation of the plan's effectiveness will be able to answer questions such as 'Have the plan's objectives been fulfilled?' 'What tasks need to be done better?' 'How effective is a specific training programme?' Besides the effectiveness we also need to measure how well (efficiently) things are being done. Thus one evaluates the current processes in use (process evaluation) as well as the outcomes and the results of the action taken (outcome evaluation).

What are the key components of evaluation which often get neglected?

It has recently been recognised that there are a number of key components of the effective provision of a District's health service which are frequently neglected during evaluation of District Primary Care. These are accessibility and coverage, community participation and community development, functional integration and support within the health service, feasibility in terms of cost, and quality of services. These components are crucial to the success of a health programme. Ways and means of measuring these components need to be included in all evaluations of District health activities.

WHAT ARE THE ESSENTIAL ELEMENTS OF PRIMARY HEALTH CARE WHICH NEED TO BE EVALUATED?

There are eight essential elements of Primary Health Care (PHC) which will obviously need to be evaluated (see figure 6.1). These are: food supply and nutrition, water and sanitation, mother and child health, immunisation, prevention and control of locally endemic diseases, management of common illnesses and injuries, provision of essential drugs, and community mobilisation and awareness. The way of evaluating PHC has now been made much easier because there is both a global analysis of what these essential elements entail and several country examples specifying precisely what the tasks under each of the eight elements are. Evaluation is then simply a question of identifying these tasks and then seeing to what extent these tasks are being put into practice (see tables 6.2 and 6.3).

Indicators for monitoring 'progress towards health for all' are being discussed at an international level and include indicators of health policy, socio-economic indicators, indicators of health status and indicators of health care provision (WHO, 1980). Health status indicators suggested include proportion of infants born with low birth weight, height and weight of children, proportion of pre-school children with small arm circumference, infant mortality rate, child mortality rate, under-five mortality rate, under-five proportionate mortality, life expectancy, maternal mortality rate, crude birth rate, disease-specific death rates, proportionate mortality from specific diseases, morbidity incidence and prevalence rates, and prevalence of long-term disability. Suggested indicators of provision of health care include coverage, physical accessibility, percentage of population served, socio-economic accessibility and population ratio to health personnel. In addition there has been a growing realisation of the need to find out what is happening at the 'front-line' of the health care system and to devise appropriate conceptual and analytical methods for doing this (WHO, 1981). This requires

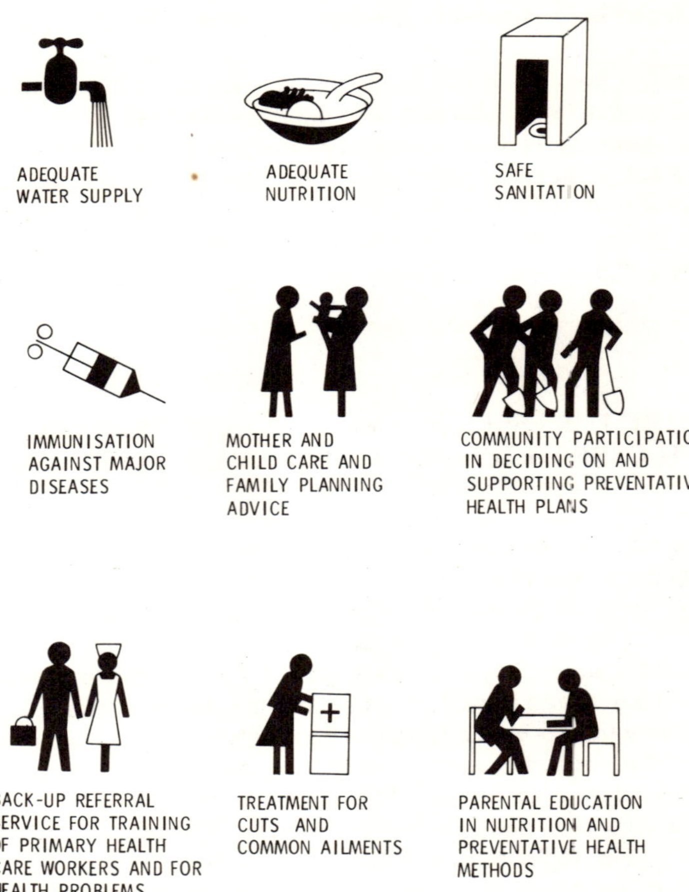

Figure 6.1   The essential elements of primary care

the orientation of front-line workers to think of disease, disability, accidents as well as vital events like pregnancy, births, deaths and so on, in terms of the total population in which they occur, the area and time in which they happen and the group of people affected. The survey method has been the mainstay of the methodology of evaluation, but it has recently come under criticism. Because of the difficulties of travel to the more remote hamlets and villages of the district, especially during the wet season, many of the rural problems go unseen. Often, survey teams do not stay overnight in the area; much of the working day is spent in travel, and during the brief period spent in the village much of their time is taken up by local reception committees. Individuals and

Table 6.2 Evaluation – what it should, can and can't do

What it should do	What it can do	What it can't do
Should come out of data collected	Use specified criteria	Can't all be done objectively. Much must be subjective
Evaluate not the project but the process of providing care		Decision-making is also based on some assessment of what is likely to work or not, usually influenced by powerful people which in turn affects results and outcome
	Indicate where change is desirable (can bring change)	Does not necessarily effect change about every item
		Cannot necessarily persuade staff to support evaluation methods and results, especially if – it is 'external' evaluation
	Give sense of direction and commitment (if done corporately)	– workers think it is 'snooping' – it appears to be threatening: people need to think some good is coming out of evaluation, otherwise will cause
	Can raise morale	disappointment or raise expectations.
	Good for training	Need to have initial hunches about what directions are possible

Table 6.3 Uses of information: good and bad

+	−
It can be of direct relevance to the work	Remove the fear that evaluation results will be used by people in authority 'up there' to criticise their work
If backed up by people with authority it helps to get things done	
Can indicate whether anything is being done about problems identified	
Can be made part of the process and not a one-off exercise	

families with problems get pushed into the background and unless a special effort is made to identify them, they are likely to go unnoticed and their problems unrecorded.

WHICH LEVEL? WHICH COMPONENT? – LEVELS OF EVALUATION (see figure 6.2)

In a District health programme several components, tasks and activities of health facilities may need evaluation. On the other hand, the evaluation may be at the level of a village, a group of villages or the entire District. Thus one may conceive of a hierarchy of evaluation, as follows:

District, health station or local community
Programme, project or local service
Components of a programme, for example, MCH, family planning, communicable disease control *or*
Comprehensive, for example, Primary Care or District Health Service
Health status, health care or determinants of ill health
Care of high risk groups

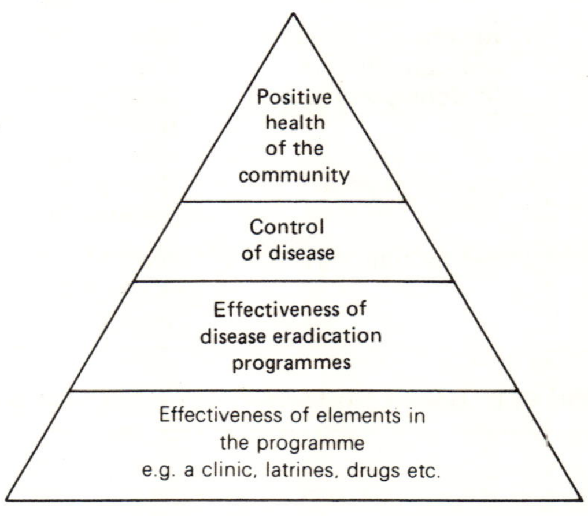

Figure 6.2   Levels of evaluation

WHAT LEVEL OF FEEDBACK AND WHICH COMPONENT IN A PROGRAMME?

Feedback can take place at a number of *different levels*; District, health station and local community to name but a few. It may focus on a programme, a project or a local service. A *single programme* may be evaluated such as mother and child care, communicable disease control, family planning, or environmental health. Alternatively there may be *comprehensive* evaluation such as of primary care or a District's over-all activities. As outlined in chapter 2, evaluation may identify the health status, the health care provision or the causes of ill health.

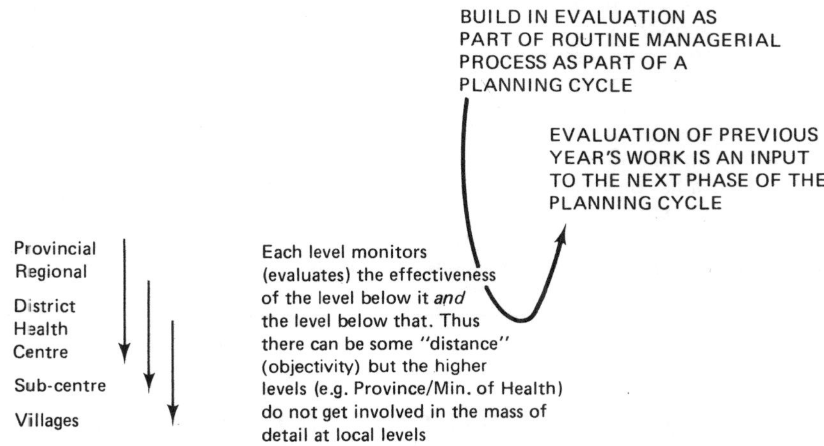

Figure 6.3   Levels of feedback and which component in a programme

WHICH SPECIFIC QUESTIONS CAN FEEDBACK FROM A HEALTH CARE PROGRAMME CONSIDER?

Feedback can consider one or two major topics out of a number of important issues. Such topics include feedback about the appropriateness and relevance of a programme, on the adequacy of services provided (this is done by comparing services with the needs for them), on effectiveness, on efficiency and on impact. Another important topic for feedback is the flexibility of a programme to respond to new directions, initiatives and needs identified while it is in progress. Acceptability of new approaches or directions can be measured with regard to the Ministry, the staff and the local people. Side effects and safety always need to be considered as well as the ethics of any feedback procedure.

HOW CAN DATA BE OBTAINED TO FIND OUT WHAT IS GOING ON?

Some of the possible sources of data have been considered in chapter 2. Other commonly listed procedures are listed in table 6.4.

Table 6.4 **Commonly listed procedures for obtaining data**

Procedure	Formal terminology
(1) Asking, talking, recording	Interviews
(2) Comparing views	Rating
(3) Watching health activities	Observing unobtrusively
(4) Writing down answers	Questionnaires
(5) Use of records	Record data analysis
(6) Use of diaries	Diaries
(7) Observing the normal flow of work	Time and motion studies
(8) Making a list of equipment and drugs consumed	Stock-taking and making inventories
(9) Discussions with community groups	Rapid rural appraisal
(10) Measuring (people, rates, specimens, foods etc.)	Surveying

QUICK OR LONG? AND WHAT DISCIPLINES IN GETTING FEEDBACK ON A PROGRAMME?

Feedback can range from 'a quick look and a good listen' to a long-term detailed investigation. It can attempt to be objective (using outsiders) or to be enlightening (when local insiders are essential). A number of disciplinary perspectives can be involved, economics (which is often quick), epidemiology and sociological (which often rely on surveys and statistical analysis), anthropological (which often requires a longer time and uses key informants for information) and political (which often relies on a non-participatory observer).

An example of 'a quick look and a good listen' is to be found in the 'community round' information described in chapter 2. The economic perspective is shown in the figures for health facilities, personnel and in the costing of salaries (all in chapter 3). Epidemiological methods show the pattern of high risk families and communities (see chapter 2), and anthropological data show for example how the women's food cropping has changed and the reasons for it (chapter 3.) Discussion with people is often necessary to supplement formal surveys and to understand the reasons why certain things are happening (see tables 6.5 and 6.6).

If information collection is to be effective then those collecting it at the local level must have a first commitment to using it themselves for decision-making, in addition to forwarding it to another level to be used by others. Thus health care providers need to learn simple methods of collection and analysis of health data so that they can act on the information they receive. It should be possible for District health staff to analyse health information using simple

Table 6.5 How is feedback done?

Quick look and listen or long term and detailed
By outsiders ('objective') or insiders ('enlightening')
Using tools of economics (usually quick, e.g. 'hard' costing of programmes and
  activities)
Using tools of epidemiology and sociology (e.g. patterns, surveys or identifying
  power groups)
Using tools of anthropology (participating observer attempting to define reasons
  for certain events)
Using tools of political science (non-participant observer)

**Table 6.6 What specific questions need to be answered for proper
feedback?**

Questions	*Comparison*
Appropriateness and relevance	Comparison with policy (chapters 2 & 3)
Adequacy, quantity and cost	Comparison with needs (chapters 2 & 3)
Effectiveness	In meeting aims (chapter 3)
Efficiency	In working methods
Impact	On specific problems
Progress flexibility	In relation to new requirements
Acceptability	To local people, to staff & to Ministry
Accessibility and distribution	Of services in relation to population and tasks to be done
Side effects and safety	
Ethics of service provision and of evaluation	
Is the feedback being evaluated?	
– how much will it cost?	
– what is unsaid?	
– what is unwritten?	
– how narrow or comprehensive is it?	
– are the results discussed?	
– with whom?	
– why are those specific people doing an evaluation?	

arithmetic (and pocket calculators if available) so that it is not necessary to
send information to national computer centres for analyses which may take
years and which will yield results long after such information has ceased to be
useful for corrective action. At present much health information gathered is
put away without being processed because the people who collect the
information cannot find immediate use for it.

EXAMPLES OF DATA COLLECTION FORMS AND SYSTEMS USED IN LOCAL COMMUNITIES

Some local community workers may like to use illustrated data collection sheets as shown in this example from Kenya (see figure 6.4). Others may like to use the wooden compartmentalised box and colour counters used in Papua New Guinea, or use the tally sheets as in Tanzania (see figure 6.5).

Records can be designed so they can be marked by non-literate people or filled in with the help of a schoolchild who can read or write.

Traditional birth attendants (TBAs) can also be taught to use coloured marbles representing well-defined and easily identifiable clinical conditions associated with pregnancy and delivery and to drop these into a container as and when such clinical conditions arise. In the Danfa Project in Ghana, traditional birth attendants have used cards of specified colours to refer patients with complications of pregnancy to midwives at health centres. TBAs can also record live births with a grain of maize dropped in a jar and stillbirths with a pebble put in a jar.

CHOICE OF EVALUATION METHOD

Experiment design, using experimental and control groups Experimental group gets programme, Control group does not

Experimental Model

	Before	*After*
Experimental	a	b
Control	c	d

If difference between a and b is greater than difference between c and d, then programme is a success. The greater the difference the more successful the programme.

Quasi-experimental design

This does not require strict adherence to the principles of the experimental design.

This is a more practical way of evaluating a programme but one must control for external factors (or variables) likely to influence the evaluation. Some examples:

(a) *Time series design*

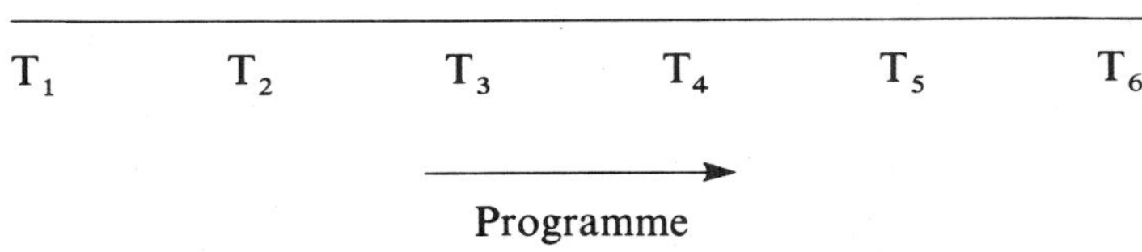

Information is collected at specified periods during the course of implementation of the programme, and all changes are noted. The assumption made is that all changes and improvements are attributable to the programme. The pitfall of course is that changes may occur as a result of the mere passage of time.

(b) *Multiple time series*

This is similar to (a) above except that the observations are made at several centres where similar health programmes are being implemented.

(3) *Non-Experimental Design*

Three examples are:
(a) Before and after – study of a single programme
(b) After only
(c) After only with a control group.

Patient care evaluation

There are three common methods which one can use to assess or evaluate the quality of care which a health institution provides for its patients. These are:

(1) *Structure* of the institution viz.
    (a) Staff
    (b) Equipment
    (c) Buildings and so on.
The limitation of this method of evaluation is that the mere presence of staff, equipment and building does not guarantee access and availability, even though the better the facilities the better the quality of care.

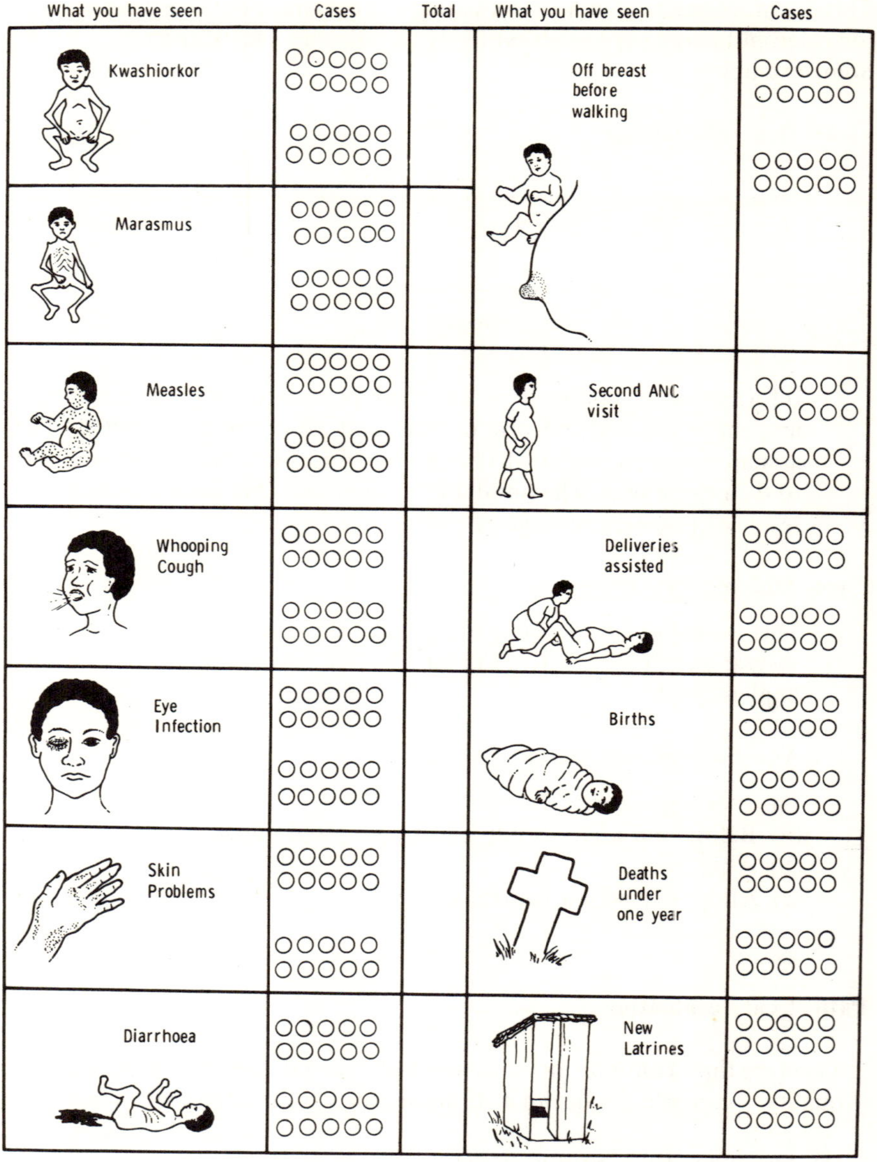

What you have seen	Cases	Total	What you have seen	Cases
Kwashiorkor			Off breast before walking	
Marasmus				
Measles			Second ANC visit	
Whooping Cough			Deliveries assisted	
Eye Infection			Births	
Skin Problems			Deaths under one year	
Diarrhoea			New Latrines	

(2) *Process.* Here the results of interactions between patients and workers are observed either directly or reviewed by means of clinic records. This type of approach is more reliable because contact between providers of care and clients is an indicator of the type and quality of the health activity.

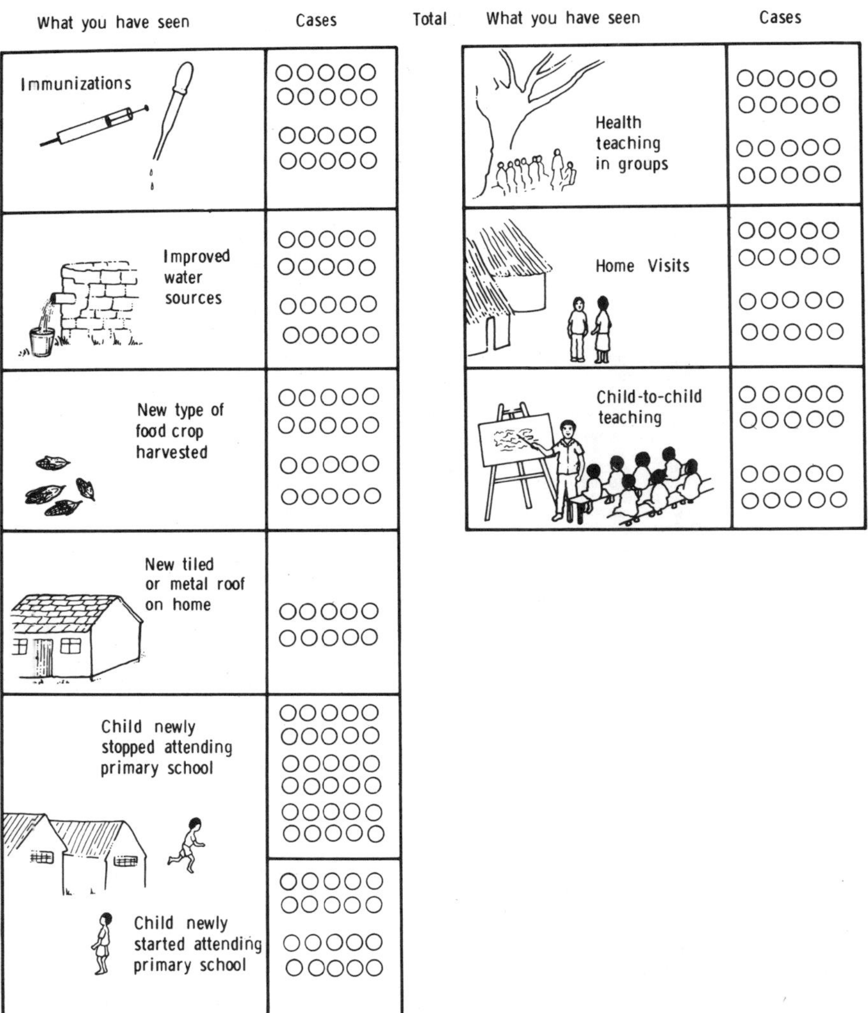

Figure 6.4   Data collection sheets for use by village health workers in Kenya

Source: Adapted from Schaffer, AMREF, Kenya.

(3) *Outcome.* This monitors changes of the health status of the patients and the community which may be attributable to programmes carried out by health institutions serving the community. This only pays off at a high level, for example, National or Regional, and over a long time scale.

District Health Care

MOTHER AND CHILD HEALTH CLINIC

Name of clinic ____ Date __________

A T T E N D A N C E

CHILDREN

FIRST ATTENDANCE

00000	00000	00000		
00000	00000	00000	Total	
00000	00000	00000		
00000	00000	00000		
00000	00000	00000		_____

THIRD ATTENDANCE

00000	00000	00000	00000	00000	
00000	00000	00000	00000	00000	Total
00000	00000	00000	00000	00000	
00000	00000	00000	00000	00000	
00000	00000	00000	00000	00000	_____

SECOND ATTENDANCE

00000	00000	00000		
00000	00000	00000	Total	
00000	00000	00000		
00000	00000	00000		
00000	00000	00000		_____

FOURTH AND SUBSEQUENT ATTENDANCE

00000	00000	00000	00000	00000	
00000	00000	00000	00000	00000	Total
00000	00000	00000	00000	00000	
00000	00000	00000	00000	00000	
00000	00000	00000	00000	00000	_____

MOTHERS

FIRST ATTENDANCE

00000	00000	00000		
00000	00000	00000	Total	
00000	00000	00000		
00000	00000	00000		
00000	00000	00000		_____

THIRD ATTENDANCE

00000	00000	00000	00000	00000	
00000	00000	00000	00000	00000	
00000	00000	00000	00000	00000	
00000	00000	00000	00000	00000	
00000	00000	00000	00000	00000	_____

SECOND ATTENDANCE

00000	00000	00000		
00000	00000	00000	Total	
00000	00000	00000		
00000	00000	00000		
00000	00000	00000		_____

FOURTH AND SUBSEQUENT ATTENDANCE

00000	00000	00000	00000	00000	
00000	00000	00000	00000	00000	Total
00000	00000	00000	00000	00000	
00000	00000	00000	00000	00000	
00000	00000	00000	00000	00000	_____

I M M U N I Z A T I O N

CHILDREN

BCG

00000	00000	00000	00000	00000	00000	00000	00000	Total
00000	00000	00000	00000	00000	00000	00000	00000	_____

SMALLPOX

00000	00000	00000	00000	00000	00000	00000	00000	
00000	00000	00000	00000	00000	00000	00000	00000	_____

DPT

1st Injection			2nd Injection			3rd Injection		
00000	00000		00000	00000		00000	00000	
00000	00000	Total	00000	00000	Total	00000	00000	Total
00000	00000		00000	00000		00000	00000	
00000	00000		00000	00000		00000	00000	
00000	00000	_____	00000	00000	_____	00000	00000	_____

POLIO

1st Dose			2nd Dose			3rd Dose		
00000	00000		00000	00000		00000	00000	
00000	00000	Total	00000	00000	Total	00000	00000	Total
00000	00000		00000	00000		00000	00000	
00000	00000		00000	00000		00000	00000	
00000	00000	_____	00000	00000	_____	00000	00000	_____

MEASLES

00000	00000	00000	00000	00000	00000	00000	00000	_____

MOTHERS

TETANUS

1st Injection			2nd Injection			3rd Injection		
00000	00000		00000	00000		00000	00000	
00000	00000	Total	00000	00000	Total	00000	00000	Total
00000	00000		00000	00000		00000	00000	
00000	00000		00000	00000		00000	00000	
00000	00000	_____	00000	00000	_____	00000	00000	_____

	I L L N E S S E S D I A G N O S E D							
MALNUTRITION	00000 00000 00000 00000 00000	00000 00000 00000 00000 00000	00000 00000 00000 00000 00000	00000 08000 00000 00000 00000	00000 00000 00000 00000 00000	00000 00000 00000 00000 00000	00000 00000 00000 00000 00000	Total
DIARRHOEA	00000 00000	00000 00000	00000 00000	00000 00000	00000 00000	00000 00000	00000 00000	
MEASLES	00000	00000	00000	00000	00000	00000	00000	
'AT RISK'	00000 00000	00000 00000	00000 00000	00000 00000	00000 00000	00000 00000	00000 00000	
RAISED BLOOD PRESSURE	00000	00000	00000	00000	00000	00000	00000	
ANAEMIA	00000	00000	00000	00000	00000	00000	00000	
FIRST ATTENDANCE IN THIRD TRIMESTER	00000	00000	00000	00000	00000	00000	00000	
'AT RISK'	00000	00000	00000	00000	00000	00000	00000	

(Left margin labels: CHILDREN for the first group of rows; MOTHERS for the lower group.)

Figure 6.5 Tally sheets for data collection for use by village health workers in Tanzania

WHO IS TO OBTAIN THE FEEDBACK INFORMATION?

Each type of person who obtains feedback information has advantages and problems. In the past much health care evaluation was done by outside consultants who had the skills and no vested interest nor commitment. Moreover, often they hardly knew the country at all, although in time some became much in tune with a particular country's needs and wishes. Nationals from another part of the country may feel just as strange as foreigners in some areas and this can cause problems.

Policy makers and planners often evaluate health care. Their problem is that they are asked to criticise their own plans and sometimes this can be difficult. However, they often do have a good overview. Programme staff and managers working on a particular project also find it difficult to be objective in evaluation. Although they may know very well what defects and deficiencies exist, they may be unable to write about them in case they lose their jobs.

Members of the community may seem to have fewer vested interests in a project yet in many countries certain factions of a community dominate health care programmes. The question is 'Who in the community should evaluate the programme and how can one section of the community be compared with another?' Academics and research staff now do health care evaluation in most countries. They can cause problems for health care personnel because their approach is sometimes too theoretical and academic and often they have little experience of working in remote areas. They may take too long to produce their reports and may not be willing or able to take decisions on what needs to be done. Another risk is the question of whether people doing evaluation should be specialists and if specialised, in what discipline. Although the choice is wide, it is usually easy to decide who is to do the evaluation provided it is clear why evaluation is needed, and what the subject is (see table 6.7).

Table 6.7 **Who is to carry out the evaluation?**

Type of person	*Advantages*	*Disadvantages*
Outside consultants	No vested interests. Will teach new skills to local workers	Sometimes do not know local situation well
Policy makers and planners	Good overview	Difficult to criticise their own plans
Programme staff and managers	Intimate knowledge of the local situation and of working with the programme	May be unwilling to be critical
Community leaders	Project often has the stated aim of serving the community	Leaders may not be truly representative
Poor groups in the community	Project aims to serve the poor	Other groups in the community may obstruct or influence them
Academics and research staff	Usually skilled in the techniques and willing to teach	May take too long to produce the report and raise too many questions
Those working in the project	Immediate feedback. Strengthens the workers' sense of responsibility for their own projects. A natural part of the management process of setting targets, implementation, supervision and control	Requires effective managers and an appropriate managerial system

WHERE SHOULD THE FEEDBACK BE DONE?

What area? What population? What sub-groups?
These are crucial questions in many districts where there is a diversity of people, health problems, and health care provision. The biases that can occur in visiting only villages near the tarmac road and talking only to élite male informants are well known and have already been referred to.

WHEN SHOULD FEEDBACK INFORMATION BE OBTAINED?

Which season of the year is selected for an evaluation to be done will influence the pattern of disease found, how effectively health personnel are able to do their work, whether the community is very busy from dawn to dusk, and therefore absent from their homes, or available to talk in a slightly less busy time. Many evaluations have been done in a short cool or dry season ignoring the fact that a country may be hot and wet for most of the time. Whatever period is chosen for an evaluation will influence what is found.

CONSTRAINTS ON GETTING FEEDBACK

The main constraints usually felt in evaluation are shortages of time, money and staff. A further major problem may occur if the evaluation is not wanted by staff or community or if the information is thought to be wanted for political reasons. If an external agency funds an evaluation it may well impose constraints. The final constraint is that evaluation always requires some effort. People will lose interest in evaluation if they do not see that it leads to changes, or confirms and encourages their current efforts.

FURTHER READING

Cole-King, S., *Approaches to the evaluation of maternal and child health care in the context of primary health care*, WHO, Geneva, HSM/79.2, 1979.
World Health Organization, *Development of Indicators for Monitoring Progress towards Health for All by the Year 2000*, WHO, Geneva, 1981.
World Health Organization, *Health Programme Evaluation*, WHO, Geneva, 1981.

7 Future Prospects: Challenges for Change

The World Health Organization has identified 'Health for all by the year 2000' as a major objective, and as part of this drive the water development decade is already upon us. Throughout the 1980s we are likely to see many changes in national policies and strategies for provision of health care in most countries. Developing countries in particular face major challenges because it is not very long ago since a joint UNICEF/WHO study pointed out that not more than 20 per cent of the rural populations in the Third World receive basic health care on a regular basis; and the plight of the urban poor is even worse despite their proximity to large medical centres. Hence most of the developing world governments face the almost impossible task of expanding health services four-fold within a decade or so. Obviously this cannot happen along the existing pattern. Many of the reasons have been discussed in previous chapters, including the inappropriateness of the existing pattern of services to national needs. A growing number of countries have realised this and are responding to the challenge by developing their own strategies for spreading primary health care. However, they face several difficulties. There is the constant problem of inadequate resources. In a world-wide recession with a large number of countries being unable even to service international loans, a cut-back on expenditure is the only policy open to most. Health services are among the first to experience cuts. Secondly, most developing countries depend upon imported drugs and equipment for their health services, and the rising costs of these items as well as deteriorating reserves of foreign exchange means acute shortages or having to do without essential supplies for many health programmes.

On the other hand, people's expectations are rising. Many have read reports of miracle drugs and heard about new techniques in surgery and in medical practice. The inability of their governments to provide such facilities in the country is taken as an admission of failure. Only a few have heard about Primary Health Care and have experienced the marked improvements in health when the water supply is made safe, when essential drugs are made available at each village, or when all the children have been immunised. Hospital specialists and consultants who dominate the health care systems in most countries are not likely to agree easily to the shift of emphasis in national health plans from hospital-based services to primary care within the community. Hence the urgent need for establishing links between community-based (level A) care and hospital (level C) services, the former utilised not as a source of 'interesting' cases but as the true front line of the health care system. Such a change is even more necessary in the towns and the cities where up to a quarter of the population may be new migrants living in the peri-urban shanty towns. The conflicting interests of the various levels of health care systems, with each level demanding ever more resources from a national budget that is shrinking in real terms, is likely to create a situation where PHC for the rural and urban poor may degenerate into a poor type of care. The solution lies in earmarking separate funds and resources for primary care, formulating sound policies and strategies, setting up training programmes, and evolving methods of learning from experience.

Encouraged by the success of the smallpox eradication programme, the World Health Organization has launched several global programmes like, for example, the expanded programme of immunization (EPI), oral rehydration therapy (ORT), promotion of breast feeding, the water and sanitation decade and so on. These programmes need to be integrated into the national strategy for PHC and may well provide the springboard for other activities in primary care. The administrative, logistical, technical and managerial needs of the above programmes will be a major part of the future challenges facing the health services of most countries. In addition, there are several trends which have evolved during the past decade and which are now being adopted internationally. The most widespread amongst these is the utilisation of health workers with less than the conventional period of professional training. There are several categories of such auxiliary health workers and different countries have adopted different standards depending upon their needs. They vary from physicians' assistants, med-exes and nurse practitioners to medical assistants, rural medical aides and maternal and child health aides. Moreover, semi-literate or illiterate community health volunteers are now increasingly becoming part of the national strategies for provision of health care, so that village health workers (VHW) and trained birth attendants (TBA) are to be found in many countries. In the average district of a developing country there are likely to be between 40 to 80 auxiliary health workers and between 100 to 200 VHWs and TBAs. They are being considered as the front-line workers or the grass-roots of the health system by national planners. The task of providing them with logistical and technical support is immense and will require considerable managerial skills. Besides, they need to be carefully integrated into the chain of health facilities and the network of health care. Their training needs are also likely to be many and varied, and require careful study. Any service is completely dependent upon the quality of its personnel. A sound policy for development of health manpower is necessary to deal with morale at all levels.

Other trends and innovations are all linked to the above trend of utilising less trained health workers. Because of their short training and background of education, their armamentarium of drugs has to be limited, and restricted to the common illnesses. Partly on account of this and partly due to economic reasons, many countries have drawn up a list of essential drugs. The managers of the District Health Teams will be continuously faced with the task of deciding between getting essential supplies to the front-line workers and procuring sophisticated equipment or expensive medicines for the hospital consultants. If hospitals are allowed to deprive front-line workers of their basic tools, then PHC will exist only on paper, and some demarcation of funding is therefore necessary. Thirdly, in the drive to simplify medical care many standardised techniques have evolved like the arm band for measuring arm circumferences, the Hyderabad-mix and similar other multi-mixes as weaning foods, the oral rehydration spoon and so on. Such new developments need to be communicated to health workers at all levels of care and so systems for communication of new ideas will have to be evolved. Programmes of distance teaching for the front-line workers in order to provide continual in-service training may need to be considered as part of the managerial process.

MANAGEMENT ISSUES LIKELY TO ARISE DURING THE NEXT DECADE

Four major management issues are apparent from the analysis of plans for Primary Health Care. These are: the need for support of teams at Level B (the Health Station); the need to solve the already existing Level B problems so that they are not perpetuated into Primary Health Care (Level A); the need to find alternative approaches to problems of accessibility and coverage; and the need to set priorities for local community (Level A) health tasks to be done.

It is obvious from the detailed analysis of workload and responsibilities that the Health Centre and sub-centre (Level B) teams are being asked to become a major pivot point in the proposed PHC system. They will need to be recognised as such in this important role and considerable support is likely to be needed for their work. Training, supplies, supervision and morale boosts are needed. Will they be forthcoming?

Unless the existing problems at Level B are solved they are likely to be perpetuated into the new Primary Health Care system. New community work commenced before facing up to and solving outstanding current rural health problems will very soon be ineffective. If, for example, a midwife at Level B does not know the importance of recognising high risk pregnancies she will have difficulty in supervising referral of such high risk pregnancies to her by the traditional birth attendant. Clearly, once such a problem is recognised, it means that midwives already in the post need to be given refresher training first, before the TBA training programme starts. But will such health care problems at present existing in the health care system be recognised? Will action be taken to solve them or will they be extended further into the system and perpetuated when PHC activities are initiated?

Calculations of expected accessibility by communities to the components of the Primary Health Care system have been made. The limiting factor is rightly recognised as travelling time from the home to the source of health care. A local community service is needed within 15 minutes of travel for everyone. Where walking is the common mode of transport such a service needs to be within one mile. The next more sophisticated level of service needs to be within one hour's travel. If walking, this should be not more than 5 miles (8 km) away. Hospital services need to be within 4–5 hours travel (to enable, for example, an emergency caesarian section in good time for an obstructed labour). This will need to be within 25 miles (40 km) assuming that emergencies and very ill patients will be carried by vehicular transport. This, of course, makes no allowance for being caught in traffic jams. Clearly, as transport methods change health service accessibility changes. Although an optimistic view suggests that mechanised transport could become available to more people through good public transport systems, more taxis or an increased number of private cars, it is also probable that in many countries fewer people will be able to travel by motorised vehicle or by animal transport because the cost has become too high.

With varying accessibility, health workers have varying degrees of responsibility for populations 'covered' by their services. Health workers need to have a specified catchment area that they are serving; yet as population movements change, the population coverage also needs to change with it.

Another problem with accessibility is that in sparsely-populated areas there may be relatively few people living within one mile (1.6 km) radius (Level A), or five-mile (8 km) radius (Level B). In the same country there may be a very large population in a one mile (1.6 km) radius in the squatter area of the capital city and very few in a mountainous region. If communities with population densities of less than 200 people in a one-mile (1.6 km) catchment area are excluded, whole sections of the poorest parts of a country are likely to be left out. How are health services to be provided in these sparsely populated areas? Clearly different options are needed. In a very densely populated area it may be efficient to have several 'specialised' workers, for example, in mother and child health care, environmental health, community development and so on. In a sparsely-populated area, it is far more likely that a multi-purpose worker will be needed who can do the more important tasks in each of these four specialities. National broadcasting stations can be persuaded to broadcast health programmes at specified times with multi-purpose workers in remote communities acting as local discussion leaders. Such an approach has been successfully tried in Lesotho and Tanzania.

Overall, recognition of these four major management issues draws attention to the options available for making progress towards health for all by the year 2000. These include:

(1) Aiming to provide a network of local community (Level A) health development posts and supportive services as well as training from the district hospitals as outlined in the plan in chapter 3.
(2) Aiming to spread Level B Health Centre/sub-centre services by extending existing services so that units are available at five mile (8 km) intervals and at the same time solving existing managerial or administrative problems as well as encouraging outreach services. Such services may also serve as means for commencing a dialogue with local communities.
(3) Aiming to strengthen Level C elements of the strategy by emphasising support and logistic services; integrated intersectoral approaches and in-service training; co-ordination with the District Council; and team work between the doctors, public health staff, health administration and environmental health, with regular planning, monitoring and evaluation of health activities.
(4) Focusing on communicable disease control, Mother and Child Health services and environmental hygiene at every level.
(5) Aiming to teach specified Level A tasks to school teachers; for example, rehydration for diarrhoea, malaria prophylaxis, measuring malnutrition, accident prevention and so on.
(6) Aiming to make the more important among Level A skills as part of the general knowledge of everyone during the coming decade through adult education, school education and the use of mass media.
(7) A combination of any of the above.

OBSTACLES AND CONSTRAINTS

Several difficulties which may impede progress towards health for all by the year 2000 also need to be recognised. The most important of these is the question of a national will. The creation of a national will for rural health care and upliftment is not a matter of issuing directives or decrees, but one of a national dialogue at all levels. And this kind of awakening is still lacking in many countries. Then there is the perennial problem of finance. When there is a high inflation rate in Europe and America, it is several times worse in many developing countries. Inflation rates of 40 to 50 per cent and even higher have been recorded for several countries. Resources in real terms may be diminishing at a time when more resources are needed. Political problems may also rear their heads. Confronted with all these difficulties, how real is the government commitment to health for all? Will lip-service, political rhetoric and grandiose policy be backed up by real resources and action? Will there be changes in curricula to provide appropriate training, for doctors and nurses as well as other types of health workers? Will career structures reflect this new training? Within the health care system will special roles and experiences be well utilised, for example, Will those who have worked in isolated places for many years to help patients with leprosy, tuberculosis or mental illness be included as trainers? Is there really any hope of improving procurement and distribution of dressings and drugs? At the local level, will the local political structure be a constraint to community development? Will the special problem of disparities in the cities be recognised, for example, the shanty towns with only token services on the one hand and the larger hospitals rapidly consuming health care resources on the other? Will the social distance between most health workers and their communities remain so great that true 'community involvement' is impossible as health workers fail to comprehend and respect the local culture in their area?

OPPORTUNITIES FOR FUTURE GROWTH

There are potential problems but there is also considerable hope. Under-used resources exist as well as unsolved problems (see table 7.1).

Already many international agencies (for example, the World Bank) are looking on health as a productive asset not a cost. It is likely that government bureaucracies will come to recognise this point of view and health will receive higher priority in national expenditure.

Never before has there been so much opportunity to share health knowledge so quickly with people around the world. The information technology revolution is only just beginning. The possibilities of improving training programmes, running frequent refresher courses, enabling continuous education and providing primary and functional adult literacy for everyone are no longer remote. Satellites, radio, television, and listening groups using learning packages, have the potential for helping people take care of themselves better, look after their surroundings and remove hazards to health, and be able to make better use of the health care system.

The disease care system in all countries complains of lack of resources and of difficulties in obtaining modern equipment and drugs. But perhaps the real challenge is to use available resources better. In many countries the large majority spend part of their wealth (in cash or as gifts) to purchase treatment when they are ill. Often this is from the local herbalist or traditional practitioner, or the nearby drug store or chemist. When this expenditure has

Table 7.1 **Problems and opportunities for future plans**

Problems	*Opportunities*
Distribution, logistics, communications	Community-based distribution utilising the successful methods of commercial organisations and businesses
Poor use of health personnel	Updating training and continuous education, distance teaching
Community health workers seem to need teaching the most elementary topics	Improve the basic education of everyone via primary schools, mass media, child-to-child activities
Health care seems to be a continuous, ever-growing burden to society.	Take more action on the social causes of ill health, poverty, environmental hazards, etc.
Lack of community health personnel	Training and career structure needed for doctors, nurses and others; integration of traditional care providers like traditional healers, birth attendants etc. into the health care system

been studied (for example, in Botswana) it has been found to be as much as the government itself spends on disease care. Could this money be used more effectively to improve health? Could people spend more effectively on preventing ill health, by improving water supply, using safer machinery and so on? And maybe this is linked to the inadequate distribution network. If aerated drinks and baby foods can find their way to every corner of a country, why not essential drugs?

Health services in developing countries have hitherto been mainly concerned with physical disease. With greater understanding of the epidemiology of illness in the community, the high prevalence of mental illness is gradually being recognised in all countries. In many of the industrial societies where community mental health services are better organised it is estimated that one in eight amongst males and one in ten amongst females is at risk of developing mental illness at some time during life. Similar data for the developing countries are not available. But social disparities, poverty and polarisation within the society tend to be greater in the developing nations and the incidence of mental ill-health is likely to be as high as in the industrial world, if not higher. Promotion of mental health through a network of services will be a major challenge in many countries.

Another important potential growth point lies at the heart of the new concepts about health. Although many people still equate health care with disease care, some are already recognising that health is not just the absence of disease. Health is to do with adapting, it is a 'freedom from the dark seas of disease', stemming from spiritual and social well-being as well as physical health. There is a Zulu saying that a person is a reflection of the people around him. As social malaise becomes commonplace, as violence, intimidation and fear rack cities in the world, more and more 'health' is likely to be seen in terms of social well-being as well as individual physical and emotional fitness.

There is now a growing awareness of environmental hazards to health; lead pollution from car exhausts; car accident rates 300 times higher per 1000 miles in developing countries compared with the United States; inadequate industrial legislation in countries where factory building has grown faster than new rules and decrees to control their use and provide safeguards for the health of the work force; social practices precipitating ill health; and the ever growing awareness that if poverty could be ameliorated, much ill health would vanish. Community development as part of action to improve health is clearly crucial. But even this will not be enough when health is seen as a dynamic entity.

THE UNTAPPED RESOURCES

Within the existing health care system one under-used potential lies in the nurses and in paramedical staff. Many have been under-utilised and under-rated for too long. Some nurses are already being given better training and appropriate career structures to fulfil their potential. Public health nurses in particular now have seven years of excellent training. In many countries they are being used very effectively to bridge community and hospital work. Physiotherapists are now being recognised as key people to help the old and disabled live as fully as possible within their community. Their in-depth training in anatomy and physiology as well as in physical therapy and aids gives them a potential to be key members of the district health team.

Perhaps there are personnel in the community who are under-utilised too; grandmothers in all societies are a main source of education in parenthood and practical child care; families in many societies still care for their elderly, the sick and the chronic sick or the terminally ill. Health care in the future can choose to build on these roles. Many societies have herbal knowledge, food preferences and taboos, and ways of looking after the sick in body or spirit. Much care within the family is never seen by the formal health care system. But when societies change and the informal system breaks down with migration or other disruptions, the formal health care system is faced with taking over such traditional roles of the family. Hence it is advisable to carefully nurture the caring and providing role of the family and strengthen it with services like home visiting and District nursing. But even when the health system does have to take on the caring and supportive functions traditionally provided by the family, there is scope for linkage. Volunteers may well come forward to help.

Often they are just those wise women and helpers in the neighbourhood who in traditional society performed similar functions and roles.

BEYOND PRIMARY HEALTH CARE?

There are always options and there will always be change. One type of Primary Health Care is certainly no panacea for all health and health care problems. As health problems change and communities become older, and if they show the increasing frequencies of chronic and degenerative disease found in the currently developed world, new patterns of health care will be needed in developing countries. They may well include the same central elements of primary health care but a system of care focused more on the old, the handicapped and chronic sick, and not, as at present, on mothers and children, the acutely ill and on prevention of communicable diseases. There will be new health care problems influenced by the political and economic situation prevailing at the time, by new training for health workers and by their perception of their roles. But if the health care system is flexible enough to monitor and respond to the changes in disease as well as changes in resources and political commitment, there could well be good health beyond the year 2000.

Index